Psychiatry Essentials for Primary Care

Psychiatry Essentials for Primary Care

Robert K. Schneider, MD, FACP
James L. Levenson, MD

AMERICAN COLLEGE OF PHYSICIANS
PHILADELPHIA

Associate Publisher and Manager, Books Publishing, Tom Hartman
Director, Editorial Production, Linda Drumheller
Developmental Editor, Victoria Hoenigke
Production Supervisor, Allan S. Kleinberg
Senior Editor, Karen C. Nolan
Editorial Coordinator, Angela Gabella
Marketing Associate, Caroline Hawkins
Cover Design, Lisa Torrieri
Index, Diane Brenner

Printed in the United States of America
Printing/Binding by Versa Press
Composition by Scribe Inc.

Library of Congress Cataloging-in-Publication Data
Psychiatry essentials for primary care / edited by Robert K. Schneider, James L. Levenson.
    p.; cm.
  Includes bibliographical references.
  ISBN 978-1-930513-71-6
 1. Psychiatry. 2. Mental illness—Diagnosis. 3. Mental illness—Treatment.
4. Primary care (Medicine) I. Schneider, Robert K. (Robert Kirwin) II. Levenson,
James L. III. American College of Physicians (2003-)
  [DNLM: 1. Mental Disorders—diagnosis. 2. Mental Disorders—therapy. WM 140
P97524 2007]

  RC454.P7824 2007
  616.89—dc22   2007025285

The authors and publisher have exerted every effort to ensure that the drug selection and dosages set forth in this book are in accordance with current recommendations and practice at the time of publication. In view of ongoing research, occasional changes in government regulations, and the constant flow of information relating to drug therapy and drug reactions, the reader is urged to check the package insert for each drug for any change in indications and dosage and for additional warnings and precautions. This care is particularly important when the recommended agent is a new or infrequently used drug.

08 09 10 11 12 / 10 9 8 7 6 5 4 3 2 1

This book is dedicated to our patients and our students, from whom we have learned so much.

*Visit http://www.acponline.org/psychessentials
for more information.*

Contents

Introduction

Case Study

Ms H is a 42-year-old woman with fatigue, headaches, and insomnia. She also has a history of "anxiety and depression." Her physical exam and initial medical work-up are essentially benign. A selective serotonin reuptake inhibitor (SSRI) was initiated and increased, but she is minimally improved.

- Is her "depression" a significant mood disorder such as major depression or dysthymia?
- Is her "anxiety" an anxiety disorder—such as generalized anxiety disorder (GAD), panic disorder (PD), obsessive-compulsive disorder (OCD), post-traumatic stress disorder (PTSD), or a phobia—or is it a manifestation of another illness?
- Was an SSRI the proper treatment choice?
- Was the SSRI given in the correct dose for an adequate length of time?
- What evidence supports these decisions?
- Does the clinician have comparable and adequate knowledge and skills to efficiently evaluate this patient's psychiatric symptoms as he or she would with another patient without nonpsychiatric symptoms?

▨ The Problems

Situations like this are occurring more frequently every day. Most patients with a psychiatric disorder who seek treatment turn to the *general* medical sector (e.g., primary care), not the *specialty* mental health sector, for care of their psychiatric disorders. In the primary care setting, however, their psychiatric disorders are frequently poorly recognized and ineffectively treated (1).

Studies consistently report that approximately 25% of primary care patients have a psychiatric disorder. Yet between 54% and 77% of these disorders will go unrecognized and untreated. Of those disorders recognized, only half will be adequately treated. Economic pressures (e.g., managed care and further deinstitutionalization of patients with chronic mental illnesses) combined with the introduction of new medications to treat psychiatric disorders have brought even more patients with psychiatric illnesses to the primary care setting. However, the clinician's time with patients is shrinking, and compensation for the work effort has diminished, while the expectation that psychiatric illnesses will be managed in the primary care setting has grown.

■ The Solutions

Scholars and practitioners alike have advocated a range of solutions that promote change in 3 broad areas: the medical system as a whole, patients' behaviors, and clinicians' clinical practice behaviors. We argue that for any changes to be effective, the clinicians' clinical practice behaviors will need to be addressed first.

Specifically, general clinicians will be required to effectively recognize, diagnose, and treat the most common mental illnesses seen in the primary care setting. If general clinicians are not proficient at these tasks, more specialized sectors of the medical care system will not function optimally and efficiently. However, many general clinicians have inadequate knowledge of psychiatric disorders, underdeveloped skills in handling them, and negative attitudes toward the treatment of patients with psychiatric disorders. Even general clinicians who have interest and significant knowledge of psychiatry, still often have gaps in their knowledge and skills. These shortcomings are problematic whether the general clinician alone treats the patient or whether he or she, in the case of more severe disorders, collaborates with a psychiatrist.

This mismatch of increased demand and insufficient psychiatric knowledge and skills has occurred in large measure because preparation during medical training has not kept pace with advances in psychiatric knowledge.

This book is designed to bring the general nonpsychiatric clinician's psychiatric knowledge and skills to the necessary level to manage psychiatric disorders in nonpsychiatric settings (e.g., primary care) efficiently and effectively. The fundamentals or essentials of psychiatry are organized and presented in this book so that the general clinician can assess and hone his or her knowledge of psychiatric disorders and their treatments. This book is *not* intended to make a general clinician into a psychiatrist nor is it intended for psychiatrists. Rather, it is intended to increase a general clinician's competency and efficiency in recognizing, diagnosing, and treating the psychiatric symptoms and disorders of his or her patients in the "de facto mental health system."

■ Goals of the Book

Psychiatry Essentials for Primary Care is designed to provide a structured overview of the most common and basic topics relevant to clinicians who see patients with psychiatric disorders in primary care settings. The following are the broad goals set forth in this book.

To enable clinicians to effectively and efficiently recognize, diagnose, and treat psychiatric illness in the primary care setting. This book is written from the point of view of the clinician in the general medical sector, particularly in primary care, who sees patients with psychiatric disorders of varying severity. For many of the patients, the clinician can properly provide treatment in the primary care setting. For some, however, referral to the specialty mental health sector and collaboration with a psychiatrist or other mental health provider will be required. This book provides guidance for both situations.

To bring the psychiatric knowledge and skills of clinicians on par with their knowledge and skills of other medical specialties. Just as a general clinician is conversant in medical specialties such as cardiology, so should he or she be conversant in psychiatry. In the case of cardiology, the general clinician should have a working knowledge of the common forms of heart disease as well as how to recognize, diagnose, and treat them. However, some of the management will be referred to or shared with a cardiologist. The same is true with psychiatry. The clinician should be able to recognize, diagnose, and treat many psychiatric disorders while referring others for collaborative specialty care.

■ Organization of the Book

The sections included in *Psychiatry Essentials for Primary Care* follow a progression from the general to the specific. In Chapter 1, we define psychiatric terms and set out the scope of the book. We review what we mean by "psychiatry" and how it pertains to primary care. Most importantly, we present an organizational matrix called **MAPSO**, designed to help organize psychiatric symptoms and disorders into an accessible and usable format. MAPSO is an acronym that stands for **M**ood disorders, **A**nxiety disorders, **P**sychoses, **S**ubstance-induced disorders, and **O**rganic or other disorders. In Chapter 2, when and how to assess the potential for suicide are discussed from the general clinician's point of view. Suicidality is conceptualized along a spectrum as opposed to a narrow focus on the relatively rare event of completed suicide.

The remainder of the book reviews specific psychiatric disorders and their treatments following the MAPSO format. The sections on mood disorders (Chapters 3 through 6) and anxiety disorders (Chapters 7 through 10) form the heart of the book. These are the psychiatric disorders most frequently seen in the primary care setting. The section on mood disorders is divided into 4 chapters that roughly follow the clinical process of recognizing, diagnosing, and then treating common mood disorders: Chapter 3, Depression: Evaluation and Case-Finding Strategies; Chapter 4, Treatment of Major Depression and Dysthymia: Initial Interventions; Chapter 5, Treatment of Major Depression and Dysthymia: What to Do When the Initial Intervention Fails; and Chapter 6, Bipolar Disorders.

The section on anxiety disorders (Chapters 7-10) is divided into 4 chapters that discuss the specific 5 anxiety disorders: Chapter 7, Panic Disorder and Generalized Anxiety Disorder; Chapter 8, Post-traumatic Stress Disorder; Chapter 9, The Phobias; and Chapter 10, Obsessive-Compulsive Disorder.

Chapter 11, The Psychoses, reviews the signs and symptoms of psychosis, the specific disorders seen by general clinicians in which psychosis is frequently present (e.g., schizophrenia, major depression, mania), and the use of antipsychotic medications.

Chapter 12, Substance Use and Psychiatric Disorders, sets forth basic concepts in addiction medicine but leaves this vast topic to other sources to cover in more detail (2). The chapter focuses on the effects and side effects of some commonly used medications or substances (e.g., corticosteroids and interferons) that can cause psychiatric disorders. Finally, we examine the interactions between comorbid substance use and psychiatric disorders, with particular focus on caffeine use, nicotine dependence, and depression.

The last section, Organic and Other Disorders, begins with Chapter 13, Cognitive (Organic) Disorders and Geropsychiatry, addresses the "**3 D's of Geropsychiatry**" (i.e., **D**ementia, **D**elirium, and late-onset **D**epression) as well as age-related cognitive changes. It also includes Chapter 14, Medically Unexplained Symptoms in Patients with Psychiatric Disorders; Chapter 15, Personality Disorders, and a final chapter (Chapter 16) on other significant psychiatric topics (Adult ADD, Eating Disorders, and Women's Mental Health) not covered elsewhere in the book.

The reader may notice several conspicuous omissions. There is no mention of childhood disorders, and neurobiology receives very little comment. Childhood disorders are mostly excluded, except for a brief discussion in the section on adult ADD, because they represent a narrow segment of general psychiatry that requires specialized knowledge and training. Neurobiology is not included because the focus of this book is clinical, and the sometimes speculative nature of neurobiology may be misleading or at least distracting from the central points of the book (3).

Each chapter in *Psychiatry Essentials for Primary Care* will reflect the following structure:

- [Name of Disorder] and the General Clinician
- Essential Concepts and Terms
- Screening or Case-Finding Strategies
- Treatment
- Key Points

[Name of Disorder] and the General Clinician

At the beginning of each chapter we attempt to capture its "theme" and the specific relevance of the topic to the general clinician. Since we have used unique approaches to some of the material, readers can use these initial sections to orient themselves and hopefully understand our point of view and approach to the subsequent material.

Essential Concepts and Terms

These sections in each chapter include both the essential or enduring concepts and the basic terminology regarding the topic of the chapter. This section covers the essential background material for the focus of the chapter (e.g., epidemiology, comorbidities, risk for suicide). As clinicians, however, we not only need to grasp the basic or essential ideas but also need to know and understand the appropriate accepted diagnostic terminology (i.e., the terms in the *Diagnostic and Statistical Manual for Mental Disorders, Fourth Edition* [DSM-IV]). Our ability to understand advances in diagnosis or treatment will depend on the knowledge of the technical terms because the scientific evidence uses these terms.

Screening or Case-Finding Strategies

The Case-Finding Strategies section focuses on the practical approach to exploring these disorders in the clinical setting with patients. The words used in conversation with patients are different than the terms in our scientific literature. With medical patients, we try to avoid technical terms like neuropathy; instead, we ask about numbness or tingling. The same is true in psychiatry. Instead of asking if the patient feels "manic," the clinician should ask the patient about a decreased need for sleep, feeling "hyper," or having a change in personality. These sections contain the "how-to" basics required to recognize and diagnose the disorders in each ensuing chapter.

Treatment

Psychopharmacology and psychotherapy are the basic treatments used for psychiatric disorders. Each of the chapters devoted to specific disorders includes a relevant treatment section. Consistent with the purpose of the book, we approach treatment considerations as general clinicians working in primary care, rather than as psychiatrists. Our recommendations regarding treatment are evidence-based where there is sufficient and reliable evidence. Case examples are included for clarification and illustration of certain points.

Key Concepts

At the end of each chapter, we list the fundamental information covered in that section. "Key Concepts" is an idea borrowed from the ACP Key Diseases book series, and we continue it here.

Notes

1. In 1978, the Epidemiologic Catchment Area Study (ECA Study), sponsored by the President's Commission on Mental Health, coined the term "de facto mental health system" in systematically documenting that most patients with a psychiatric disorder turn to the general medical sector, not the specialty mental health sector, for treatment.

2. Galanter M, Kleber HD, eds. *The American Psychiatric Publishing Textbook of Substance Abuse Treatment.* 3rd ed. Washington, DC: American Psychiatric Publishing, Inc; 2004.

3. For child psychiatry, the reader is referred to Wiener JM, Dulcan MK, eds. *The American Psychiatric Publishing Textbook of Child and Adolescent Psychiatry.* 3rd ed. Washington, DC: American Psychiatric Publishing, Inc; 2004. For more on neurobiology, the reader is referred to Schatzberg AF, Cole JO, DeBattista C. *Manual of Clinical Psychopharmacology.* 6th ed. Washington, DC: American Psychiatric Publishing, Inc; 2007.

1

Basic Concepts and Terminology in Psychiatry for Primary Care: MAPSO

■ Making Use of Psychiatric Terms and Concepts

Our goal is to enable general clinicians to be as efficient and adept at diagnosing psychiatric disorders as they are at diagnosing nonpsychiatric disorders. For example, within the first 5 minutes of most patient interactions, a practicing general clinician has usually generated a differential diagnosis and is zeroing in on the most likely cause of the symptoms. Accomplishing this degree of efficiency requires a detailed understanding of the terms and concepts needed to describe the likely disorders as well as an organizational construct for the material. This kind of thinking is an associative process (as compared to a linear or algorithmic one) that typically goes on outside the direct awareness of the clinician. During the interaction with the patient, a clinician generates a series of hypotheses (i.e., differential diagnoses) that seemingly "jump" into his or her mind while hearing the patient's symptoms; subsequently, further questions are asked to rule in or rule out specific diagnoses. These cognitive processes are not random; they are learned, practiced, and ultimately performed with innate efficiency.

A 50-year-old woman presents with acute onset of chest pain and shortness of breath. The clinician should stop for a moment and notice his or her own internal cognitive process after this short description. The components of age (50 years), gender (female), onset (acute), and symptoms (chest pain, shortness of breath) are shuffled and sorted outside of the clinician's awareness. He or she probably accesses some kind of organizational system. General categories are typically considered first, such as cardiac, pulmonary, gastrointestinal, musculoskeletal, and so on. Based on additional information from the patient, including severity, associated symptoms, or other medical conditions, the clinician will consider specific diagnoses (e.g., myocardial infarction, pulmonary embolus, esophageal reflux, intercostal muscle spasm). Then, to make a tentative diagnosis, he or she will ask very specific questions. Is it changed by exertion? Does eating affect it? Most clinicians are well versed in common diseases as well as in the terminology and questions required to separate one medical diagnosis from another. They can communicate about these diseases with a wide variety of patients in diverse situations by using various techniques that have evolved out of their cumulative practice experiences.

However, in clinical situations that warrant consideration of psychiatric diagnoses, most general clinicians do not have the same cognitive facility that they have when considering general medical diagnoses. It seems that the basic terminology and organizational constructs necessary to make efficient psychiatric diagnoses are lacking, and instead of having an efficient clinical interaction with a patient, the clinician's thought process stumbles along or is brought to a halt. The result is that psychiatric diagnoses are segregated instead of being integrated in a broad set of differential diagnoses. It is not uncommon to hear nonspecific language from clinicians, like *nervous condition* or *psych problem*, instead of specific terms, such as *recurrent major depression* or *generalized anxiety disorder*. The false dichotomy between medicine and psychiatry has lead to unfortunate statements to patients, like: "I can't find anything wrong with you, so I think your condition is caused by stress and maybe you should see a psychiatrist."

We are *not* suggesting that a general clinician must become a psychiatrist to evaluate psychiatric symptoms. Rather, general clinicians should be able to discuss common psychiatric disorders and their symptoms with patients with the same ease with which they discuss other medical conditions and have the technical language to obtain useful evidence from the literature. Most general clinicians already possess much psychiatric knowledge. However, there are gaps in their knowledge, and many of the psychiatric terms and concepts they use are nonspecific and incomplete. Further, clinicians often lack an organized, logical hierarchy of psychiatric terms and concepts. An organizational system is required to efficiently move through complex terminology and concepts in psychiatry just as in cardiology. Much like in Figure 1-1, the mind of the general clinician often has all of the terms mixed together. In "computer-speak," he or she has "all files and no folders."

The DSM-IV (*Diagnostic and Statistical Manual for Mental Disorders*, Fourth Edition), which clinicians and researchers rely on as a psychiatric reference, offers a detailed and complex hierarchy of 18 diagnostic categories that includes over 6000 signs, symptoms, and inclusion criteria. Most of the current psychiatric research and evidence bases are communicated using the terms contained in the DSM-IV. This makes sense because the DSM-IV was explicitly developed to improve communication between

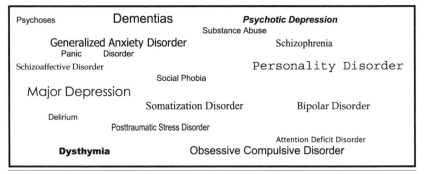

Figure 1-1

researchers and clinicians by using a consistent diagnostic system built on a descriptive approach. This descriptive or phenomenological classification system is objective and has greatly improved the reliability of psychiatric diagnoses over previously utilized subjective, theoretical, and diagnostic classifications. To utilize the growing scientific evidence base, psychiatrists have developed cognitive structures that help organize this material, but general clinicians have different needs and training. Thus, general clinicians require an organizational matrix that meets their unique clinical situations and training.

■ MAPSO: An Organizational System for Clinical Decision Making

We have developed the acronym **MAPSO** (**M**ood, **A**nxiety, **P**sychoses, **S**ubstance-induced, and **O**rganic and other disorders) to provide an organizational matrix to aid the general clinician (see Figure 1-2). MAPSO represents an integration of competing organizational concepts: major symptom categories, important etiologies, and the most common categories of psychiatric disorders seen in the general medical setting. Why 5 domains? Because the human brain cannot easily carry 18 diagnostic categories, but it can typically hold at least 5 (1,2). By using MAPSO, the general clinician has a hierarchy to organize all of those "files" of psychiatric terms and concepts into "folders" or domains with the headings mood, anxiety, psychoses, substance-induced, and organic/other. With an organizational system such as MAPSO, general clinicians can cognitively approach psychiatric disorders much as they would medical disorders (see Table 1-1).

MAPSO is a broad organizational structure of psychiatric information that is useful in *clinical* decision making for clinicians working in general medical settings. It is not a good system for psychiatrists working in specialty mental health settings because its resolution is too coarse. Accordingly, MAPSO may break down if used by a psychiatrist or mental health specialist for patients in the specialty mental health setting because it does not encompass *all* of the psychiatric knowledge needed for this specialized setting.

Most general clinicians cannot organize and access information in terms of 18 categories of equal "weight" arranged sequentially in a catalogue like the DSM-IV. Psychiatrists use psychiatric knowledge and concepts every day, so they develop their own unique recursive problem-solving strategies to efficiently consider the clinical possibilities in the 18 DSM-IV categories. However, the general medical clinician does not normally think about the full range of psychiatric information and diagnostic categories like a psychiatrist

Mood	Anxiety	Psychoses	Substance-Induced	Organic and Other

Figure 1-2

Table 1-1 MAPSO Psychiatric Organizational Matrix

Mood	**A**nxiety	**P**sychoses	**S**ubstance-Induced	**O**rganic and Other
Major Depression Single episode vs Recurrent episodes	**Generalized Anxiety Disorder (GAD)**	Schizophrenia Schizoaffective disorder	**ALL Psychoactive Substances:** Over-the-counter drugs	**Organic (due to general medical condition)** Medications
Dysthymia Minor Depression for 2 years	**Panic Disorder** **Post-traumatic Stress Disorder (PTSD)**	**Bipolar I (Mania)** Psychotic depression Dementias "Organic" psychoses (delirium)	Prescription drugs Herbal Supplements Caffeine Nicotine	Dementias HIV Traumatic brain injury
Bipolar Disorders Bipolar I Bipolar II Cyclothymia	**Obsessive-Compulsive Disorder (OCD)** **Phobias** Social Specific		Alcohol Cannabis Cocaine Opioids Stimulants **Intoxication** **Side effect** **Withdrawal** **Long-term effect**	**Other Psychiatric Illness** Personality disorder Somatization disorder Eating disorder ADHD

does, in part because a general clinician is juggling multiple diagnostic strategies and categories other than psychiatric ones. In any case, the DSM-IV is a useful resource, but it was not intended to be a rigidly applied diagnostic "bible" and was definitely not intended to be used directly as a clinical tool guiding patient interactions.

Discussing Psychiatric Symptoms with Patients

There is a myth that patients do not wish to discuss psychiatric symptoms with general clinicians. The World Health Organization (WHO) conducted a multinational, multisite study and concluded that patients were just as likely to discuss their psychiatric symptoms as their physical ones—*if asked*. Patients typically present to their general clinicians with medical symptoms (as opposed to psychiatric symptoms) because this is the patient's expectation of a typical interaction in a medical setting (3). Just because patients "typically" interact this way does not mean the patient has a latent resistance to discussing psychiatric symptoms. Perhaps it is the clinician, not the patient, who is reluctant to discuss psychiatric symptoms. Not surprisingly, the study also found that the better the relationship between the patient and general clinician, the more likely they were to discuss all symptoms, medical and psychiatric.

MAPSO provides an important cognitive tool by organizing psychiatric terms for the general clinician. This in turn makes these concepts more readily available in the clinician's working memory when addressing patients' psychiatric symptoms in a general medical setting.

What Is a Psychiatric Disorder?

A psychiatric disorder is a cluster of abnormal symptoms that persist over time and result in significant dysfunction in multiple spheres, such as personal, occupational, and social roles. The diagnostic process does not stop here; a clinical judgment is then made regarding whether or not this constellation of symptoms is in fact a psychiatric disorder. The DSM-IV is a complete listing of all psychiatric disorders and the inclusion criteria or symptoms for each disorder. The DSM-IV is an excellent system for the study of psychiatric disorders, but it has significant limitations when used to make psychiatric diagnoses in a general medical setting. First, almost all psychiatric disorders occur across a clinical spectrum as opposed to within strict categories; the DSM-IV is a catalog of categorically defined disorders. Second, the DSM-IV lists inclusion criteria and symptoms, not screening questions. The DSM-IV's clinical utility is in providing a consistent and reliable language for the study of these disorders. It is important to recall that psychiatric disorders are not diseases with clear phenotypic boundaries, and they are not defined by etiology. Medical disorders like hypertension and migraine are more analogous to psychiatric disorders than are medical diseases with clear phenotypic boundaries, like pneumococcal pneumonia or Hodgkin lymphoma.

MAPSO, in contrast to the DSM-IV, is a clinical tool that focuses on the basic symptom categories (e.g., mood/affect, anxiety, psychoses) while simultaneously addressing important etiological considerations (e.g., whether it is substance induced, "organic," or due to a general medical condition). Also, by limiting the domains to 5, clinicians can more easily hold these general domains in their "working memories" while interviewing their patients. This approach is similar to considering "organ system" etiologies (i.e., cardiac, pulmonary, gastrointestinal, musculoskeletal) with a patient complaining of chest pain.

A common mistake among both psychiatric and nonpsychiatric clinicians is the belief that if a patient has the signs and symptoms that meet DSM-IV diagnostic inclusion criteria for a particular psychiatric disorder, then the patient must have that psychiatric disorder. For example, a woman who is experiencing mood swings, tearfulness, decreased energy, weight gain, poor sleep, worry, and difficulty going to work each day may have major depression, but she may also be pregnant, perimenopausal, hypothyroid, or none of these. When a diagnosis of a psychiatric disorder is made, the patient should have the necessary inclusion criteria for that disorder. The patient seldom has *all* of the signs and symptoms of the disorder listed in the DSM-IV for that disorder, but the patient should exhibit the minimum signs and symptoms to meet the inclusion criteria for that disorder. The correlation between the patient's signs and symptoms and the DSM-IV criteria for a psychiatric disorder allows clinicians to more accurately apply the evidence from the psychiatric literature. A psychiatric diagnosis is ultimately a complex clinical judgment that occurs after a clinician assesses a patient's symptoms, the severity of the symptoms, and the degree of the patient's functional impairment. A diagnosis should always be based on the clinician's judgment, never a symptom checklist alone. This clinical judgment is primarily informed by the information obtained in an interview with the patient.

■ Screening Questions

Screening instruments such PRIME MD exist, but they are algorithmic and can be cumbersome when used in the context of a clinical interview. DSM-IV criteria are sometimes misused as screening questions, leading to jargon-laden questions such as, *Are you anhedonic?* or *Have you experienced agoraphobia?* In this book, we suggest basic screening questions for the categories of symptoms and the major psychiatric disorders contained in MAPSO. For example, the question, *Are you depressed?* is about

90% sensitive but only 57% specific for detecting a current major mood disorder (e.g., major depression, dysthymia). However, if the clinician then adds an additional question to the screening strategy about anhedonia such as, *Have you lost interest in doing pleasurable things?* then the sensitivity reaches 95%, and the specificity increases to 90%.

General Characteristics of Good Screening Questions

Discussing specific symptoms with patients requires special language and skills. To use a medical analogy, people do not intuitively know how to discuss diarrhea with other people. Clinicians learn about the disorders (e.g., diarrhea secondary to malabsorption), find valid screening processes, then develop these skills. The clinician becomes skilled at asking questions that may seem uncomfortable or unnatural to discuss, such as asking a patient with diarrhea if it awakens him at night, if is it particularly malodorous, and if is there something that looks like an oily substance in the commode (a sign of fat malabsorption). Whether discussing diarrhea or depression, some general themes arise.

- Use plain language and avoid jargon.
  What do you do for fun or pleasure? (screening for anhedonia)
- Be specific and quantify symptoms when possible.
  Let's go through a typical night. What time to you start trying to go to sleep? (exploring insomnia)
- Have a nonjudgmental stance.
  When was your last drink of beer, wine, or liquor? (instead of *Do you drink too much?*)
- Balance between open and closed questions.
  How has the depression changed things for you? (instead of either extreme: *How have you been?* or *Has the depression affected your sleep, appetite, concentration, sex drive, or willingness to be with others?*)
- Explain and then inquire.
  Some people who have major depression also experience the opposite of depression, where they have racing thoughts and feel full of energy. Have you? (screening for mania)

Screening for Psychiatric Disorders and Predictive Values

General considerations for predictive values of screening strategies for psychiatric disorders are, not surprisingly, identical to those for medical disorders. Screening, or case-finding, questions are different than diagnostic questions or instruments. If a patient answers affirmatively when asked if he or she ever has chest pain after exertion, then more specific diagnostic tests would be performed subsequently. We would not move directly to treatment based on a simple symptom report of angina alone. The same is true when working with psychiatric disorders. The question, *Are you depressed?* is very sensitive but not specific. Treatment for major depression should not be initiated with one positive screening question. A positive answer to a screening question requires further diagnostic questions, and only then should treatment be considered. The general rule is that the greater the number of symptoms present, the greater the likelihood of a disorder.

False positives to psychiatric screening questions for one psychiatric disorder may indicate that another psychiatric disorder is present. For example, a patient who answers "Yes" to *Are you depressed?* but does not have major depression (determined after asking more specific questions) may have an anxiety disorder (or another non-mood disorder), be in the early stages of a major depressive episode, or have a subsyndromal state of depression. When followed over time, patients who screen as false positives have greater impairment and utilize health care services more often than those who screen negative. The clinician should have a strategy for follow-up with patients who have false-positive screening for psychiatric disorders (4).

Screening for a Family History of a Psychiatric Disorder

Psychiatric illness in a patient's biological relatives is a strong risk factor for many psychiatric disorders. Screening for a family history adds valuable information when determining if a set of symptoms is in fact a psychiatric disorder. The utility of this approach is similar to the value of a positive family history for coronary heart disease when assessing a patient with acute chest pain. However, unlike screening for coronary artery disease, a patient may falsely or incorrectly deny a family history of a psychiatric disorder because of stigma and embarrassment or because family members with psychiatric disorders never told anyone or never sought treatment.

Using a question like, *Has any relative in your family ever had similar symptoms?* can get around initial resistance to discussion of family psychiatric history. The clinical utility of a family history is that it increases the specificity of the clinician's assessment. In other words, a positive response to screening for a psychiatric disorder in a relative of a patient increases the likelihood that a psychiatric disorder is the cause of the patient's symptoms; however, a negative family history does not significantly decrease the likelihood.

KEY POINTS

- Clinicians make clinical diagnoses quickly and accurately by recognizing patterns of symptoms and then generating hypotheses.
- This associative cognitive process often happens outside conscious awareness and requires the clinician to know and understand basic concepts and terminology involved in the disorders being considered.

- MAPSO provides a matrix that organizes fundamental psychiatric terminology for nonpsychiatrists.
- When asked, most patients discuss psychiatric symptoms as readily as physical symptoms.
- Psychiatric screening questions have comparable sensitivities to other screening tests used in medicine.
- Fluid, practical screening and diagnostic questions are the keys in the diagnostic process.
- A psychiatric disorder is a cluster of abnormal symptoms that persist over time and result in significant dysfunction in multiple spheres (i.e., personal, occupational, and social roles).
- Ultimately, it requires a clinician's judgment as to whether or not the patient's symptoms represent a psychiatric disorder.

REFERENCES

1. Miller GA. The magical number seven, plus or minus two: Some limits on our capacity for processing information. *The Psychological Review*. 1956;63:81-97.
2. Gobet F. Expert memory: a comparison of four theories. *Cognition*. 1998;66:115-152.
3. Simon GE, VonKorff M, Piccinelli M, et al. An international study of the relation between somatic symptoms and depression. *NEJM* 1999;341:1329-1335.
4. Leon AC, Portera L, Olfson M, et al. False positive results: A challenge for psychiatric screening in primary care. *Am J Psychiatry*. 1997;154:1462-1464.

KEY REFERENCES

First MB, ed. *Diagnostic and Statistical Manual of Mental Disorders*. 4th ed. Washington, DC: American Psychiatric Association; 2000.

Kendler KS. Psychiatric genetics: a methodologic critique. *Am J Psychiatry*. 2005; 162(1):3-11.

Kupfer DJM, First MB, Regier DA. *A Research Agenda for DSM-IV*. Washington, DC: American Psychiatric Publishing, Inc.; 2002.

Kendler KS. Reflections on the relationship between psychiatric genetics and psychiatric nosology. *Am J Psychiatry*. 2006;163(7):1138-1146.

Zimmerman M. *Interview Guide for Evaluating DSM-IV Psychiatric Disorders and the Mental Status Examination*. East Greenwich, RI: Psych Press Products; 1994.

2

The Spectrum of Suicidality

■ Identifying Suicidality in the Primary Care Setting

Though suicide (i.e., killing oneself) is relatively rare, suicidality (i.e., thinking about not continuing to live or ambivalence about "going on") is very common in severe psychiatric disorders. Many patients with severe psychiatric disorder are seen in general medical settings, not just specialty mental health settings. As the general clinician's knowledge and skills increase with regard to psychiatric disorders, he or she is going to detect more patients with suicidality. Keep in mind that suicidality, even if it has been neither detected nor evaluated, is often present in patients with severe psychiatric disorders. Like chest pain, suicidality can represent a genuine clinical emergency, but much more often it is not an emergency. In any case, the general clinician requires the knowledge and skills to fully assess patients with either chest pain or suicidality.

■ Epidemiology

Suicide has a base rate of 12 per 100,000 in the general population. It is estimated that a major mental disorder is present in more than 90% of suicides. This information is inherently flawed because it is collected retrospectively via "psychological autopsies" that screen for evidence of an antemortem psychiatric disorder; however, there is no alternative way to determine the rate. Of the psychiatric conditions in people who complete suicide, depression accounts for 50%, alcohol and drug abuse for 20% to 25%, and schizophrenia or bipolar disorder for 10%. These add up to more than 100% because people who commit suicide may have more than one psychiatric diagnosis. Many textbooks cite high lifetime rates of suicide in depression (15%), substance abuse (15%), and schizophrenia (10%). However, we consider these overestimates because they are based on older studies of psychiatric inpatients. More recent studies that include many outpatients suggest the risk to be much lower but still significant, with a 6% rate of suicide in depression, 7% in alcohol dependence, and 4% in schizophrenia. Other psychiatric disorders that are characterized by impulsivity, such as post-traumatic stress disorder (PTSD), panic disorder, and personality disorders, also increase the risk for suicide. In general, all psychiatric disorders carry a greater risk for suicide when compared to the general population.

◼ The Spectrum of Suicidality

Suicide attempts are possibilities in all psychiatric disorders and can be life-threatening. The term "suicide," or "completed suicide," refers to the actual act of killing oneself. However, "suicidal ideation" and "suicidality" are on a spectrum of thoughts, feelings, and ultimately actions ranging from feeling hopeless, to imagining "not being here" (e.g., going to sleep and not waking up—although not necessarily "dying"), to wishing that one could die, to planning for suicide (or self-harm), to taking actions and hurting or killing oneself.

While some thoughts or feelings on this spectrum are frequently present in severe psychiatric disorders (e.g., major depression), completed suicide is relatively rare. In the United States, it is estimated that more than 5,000,000 people will think about suicide yearly, but less than 30,000 people will actually complete suicide. Despite decades of studies documenting epidemiological correlations with suicide (i.e., risk factors), there is no effective screening approach that can be used in a clinical situation to predict suicidality; even if one screens with all recognized risk factors, there are too many false positives and false negatives. Because it is impossible to predict suicide with any reliability, the clinician's job is to fully assess the patient's suicidality and create a plan that addresses the patient's unique set of risk factors and protective factors. The risk is never zero.

Assessing for suicidality requires the clinician to discuss more than intent to commit self-harm. Hopelessness and related emotions (e.g., pessimism, negativity, demoralization) are some of the most consistent markers for severity of a psychiatric disorder, particularly a mood disorder. When assessing for suicidal ideation, it is best to start at the less severe end of the spectrum (i.e., hopelessness) and then proceed to greater degrees. By assessing potential suicidality across its entire spectrum, the clinician *and* patient gain greater insight into the severity of the underlying disorder.

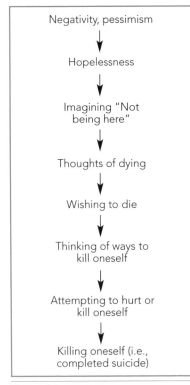

Figure 2-1

Also, patients are usually more willing to discuss hopelessness and negativity than suicide.

Screening for suicidality is similar to screening for alcoholism; asking, *Are you an alcoholic?* is abrupt and unlikely to give meaningful information. Asking, *Are you going to kill yourself?* is equally unproductive. In asking patients about suicidal ideation, clinicians should start at the less serious end of the spectrum of suicide risk. While it is critical to identify patients at the more serious end—that is, those who have a plan and are intent on carrying it out—it is also important to identify patients at lesser degrees of risk to permit earlier preventive interventions. The questions used to identify those "on the less extreme end" typically lead to very useful information regarding the *severity* of the disorder, thereby helping to uncover patients at potentially greater risk, even when those same patients honestly deny that they wanted to hurt themselves.

The hopelessness and negative thoughts engendered by many psychiatric disorders are at the core of many patients' distress and dysfunction. By determining the depth of the patient's hopelessness and helplessness (i.e., spectrum of suicidality), the clinician has obtained some of the best markers of severity. Additionally, having these symptoms validated by the clinician and targeted in treatment is exceedingly important to the patient's recovery.

The questions in Box 2-1 demonstrate a logical sequence proceeding from lower to higher risk.

This approach facilitates conversation and opens the door for further discussion when more explicit suicidal ideation is present. Some patients do not realize that simple hopelessness and despair, without thoughts about suicide, may be symptoms of a disorder. Frequently the symptoms are related to a stressor, and because the despair has a "good reason" the suicidal ideation is dis-

> **Box 2-1 Screening Questions:**
> **Spectrum of Suicidality**
>
> ---
>
> Are you having difficulty staying hopeful?
> What things in the future do you look forward to?
> Have you ever felt life isn't worth living?
> Did you ever wish you would go to sleep and not wake up?
> Have you had increased thoughts about death or dying?
> Have these thoughts ever been about taking your own life?
> Have you imagined the way you would do it?
> Are you currently considering or planning to hurt (or kill) yourself?

counted. When there is no associated stressor, patients feel they are going "crazy" because their symptoms have no logical cause. The clinician has an opportunity to educate and reassure the patient by explaining that these thoughts and feelings are symptoms of a disorder (e.g., major depression) and can be expected to go away with treatment. Especially at these times, it is helpful for the patient to understand that his or her psychiatric condition is similar to a severe medical condition and that the symptoms will

Case Study

Ms A is a 58-year-old woman with a long history of dysthymia. She comes in for an appointment because of worsening depressive symptoms. In the course of assessing the severity of her symptoms, you ask, *Are you still hopeful about the future?* She replies that she "really doesn't care much any more." You inquire further with, *How bad does it get?* She then replies, "Well, I'd never kill myself, but I wouldn't mind if God brought me home."

In this example, the clinician would not have uncovered the full extent of her current thoughts and symptoms if he or she had only asked the single question, *Are you going to kill (hurt) yourself?* The patient would have honestly answered no. The fuller communication gained from initially approaching suicidality broadly gives additional information about the severity of the disorder, the presence or absence of protective factors for suicide, as well as diagnostic information. The example of Ms A will be elaborated throughout this chapter.

resolve much like pain in rheumatoid arthritis will decrease with anti-inflammatory drugs.

■ Suicide Risk Assessment

Explicit and direct discussion about suicidal intent takes place *after* the gradual approach outlined above if suicidal thoughts are present. Pursuing details of the suicidal thoughts (e.g., onset, frequency, method, lethality of method, specificity of plan, access to means) helps the clinician establish the intensity of the suicidal ideation. It is critical to ask any patient with the potential for suicidality about his or her access to firearms. The additional questions in Box 2-2 are examples that may be helpful.

Box 2-2 Example Questions: Suicide Risk Assessment
When did you first notice these thoughts?
Are they constant or episodic (off and on)?
Have these thoughts progressed to any plans?
Have you taken any steps to advance these plans?
Have you acted on these thoughts?
Do you have access to any guns?

Next, to counterbalance the suicidal thoughts of the patient, the clinician should discuss the patient's reasons for living. It is helpful to look actively for future plans, people to support the patient, and direct prohibitions to suicide (e.g., religious beliefs). These questions often help patients approach their suicidal ideations from perspectives they may not have considered. The questions in Box 2-3 illustrate this approach:

Box 2-3 Example Questions: Prohibitions to Suicide

What keeps you from acting on these thoughts?
Who can help you through this difficult time?
What future plans do you have?
How would your death impact the people around you?

Case Study—Continued

Ms A is a 58-year-old woman with a long history of dysthymia. She comes in for an appointment because of worsening depressive symptoms. In the course of assessing the severity of her symptoms, you ask, *Are you still hopeful about the future?* She replies that she "really doesn't care much any more." You inquire further with, How bad does it get? She then replies, "Well, I'd never kill myself, but I wouldn't mind if God brought me home."

In this example, the clinician would not have uncovered the full extent of her current thoughts and symptoms if he or she had only asked the single question, *Are you going to kill (hurt) yourself?* The patient would have honestly answered no. The fuller communication gained from initially approaching suicidality broadly gives additional information about the severity of the disorder, the presence or absence of protective factors for suicide, as well as diagnostic information. The example of Ms A will be elaborated throughout this chapter.

When Is Deliberate Self-harm Not a Suicide Attempt?

Deliberate self-harm (DSH) is common in nonclinical and clinical populations. Because it is typically done secretly and not reported, often no one is aware of it. One recent study in military recruits reported that approximately 4% had a lifetime history of DSH (1). Deliberate self-harm is particularly associated with borderline personality disorder (BPD), which is the only diagnosis in the DSM-IV that includes deliberate self-harm in its description, though DSH has been found in patients with anxiety disorders (particularly PTSD), substance abuse, eating disorders, and schizophrenia. Skin cutting (70%) is by far the most common form of DSH, followed by banging or hitting oneself (21%-44%) and skin burning (15%-35%). When a clinician discovers DSH in a patient, assessment for suicidality is essential, but frequently no suicidal intent is present. Referral for a full psychiatric assessment is recommended, but if the patient is not actively suicidal or otherwise dangerous, outpatient evaluation is reasonable.

Risk Factors

Risk Factors for Completed Suicide

When genuine, significant risk for suicide is discovered, it is clinically useful to categorize the risk along 4 dimensions:

1. Chronic/predisposing factors that affect lifetime risk for suicide
2. Acute/potentiating factors that occur in immediate proximity to suicidality
3. Protective factors that, when present, mitigate against acute or chronic risks and, when absent, increase risk
4. Lethality of the suicide plan

A clinician's skills in assessing the spectrum of suicidality and accurately categorizing suicide risk are essential for managing patients with psychiatric disorders (see Table 2-1). These skills are analogous to the skills required to assess chest pain and its nuances. Most chest pain does not represent a myocardial infarction. A clinician should not send all patients with chest pain to the emergency room for thrombolytics, nor should he or she send all patients with suicidal ideation to the emergency room for admission.

Table 2-1 Risk Factors for Suicide

Chronic/ Predisposing	Acute/ Potentiating	Protective	Lethality
Male	Recent extreme	Marriage	Likelihood of
Older age (>65	loss	Religious affiliation	death (i.e.,
years)	Exacerbation of	Children in the	potential lethality
White or Native	a psychiatric	household	of means)
American	disorder	Positive social	Access to means
Prior suicide	Exacerbation of	support	Extent/details of
attempt	a medical		plan
Psychiatric	condition		Attempt where
disorder	Impulsivity		unlikely to be
Chronic medical	Access to firearms		discovered
condition	Substance abuse		
Family history	High lethality of		
of suicide	suicide plan		
Chronic pain			
Substance abuse			

■ Chronic/Predisposing Risk Factors for Suicide

Chronic/predisposing risk factors are fixed and therefore establish a base-line risk for suicide. The most studied predisposing epidemiologic factors are gender, race, and age. Men are at least 4 times more likely to commit suicide than women. However, women are about 10 times more likely to attempt suicide or make suicidal gestures. Whites and Native Americans have significantly higher suicide rates than African Americans, Hispanics, or Asians. In the United States, white men commit 73% of suicides. Age is also a significant risk factor. Suicide rates start dramatically increasing in the sev-enth decade of life, especially for men.

Prior suicide attempts represent a significant increased risk for a subse-quent attempt and for future completed suicide. A prior suicide attempt of any description is associated with an almost 40-fold increase in suicide risk-greater than the increased risk associated with any psychiatric disorder.

The presence of a psychiatric disorder can pose acute or chronic risk for suicide depending upon the patient's past history and the acuity of the symptoms. When inactive symptoms of the disorder (i.e., during remission or recovery) are reactivated (i.e., during relapse or recurrence), the chron-ically elevated baseline risk for suicide is acutely increased. Knowing where the patient falls longitudinally within the progression of their disorder also helps the clinician assess risk. For example, patients early in the course of schizophrenia carry a greater risk than those later in the course. Most sui-cides (60%) in people who have schizophrenia occur within 6 years of the first hospitalization. Substance abuse, especially severe alcoholism, is a chronic risk factor. For some alcoholics in later life, when the social effects of chronic use have accumulated (e.g., isolation, alienation), a sudden or signif-icant change (e.g., medical disease, divorce, loss of a job, death of loved one) carries a particularly high risk for suicide. On the other hand, alcohol intoxi-cation is an acute risk that quickly passes after the patient is sober.

Patients with a chronic high risk for suicide should be managed in con-cert with a psychiatrist. For example, a patient may have a long history of multiple drug overdoses with subsequent psychiatric hospitalizations. This patient will most likely have suicidal ideation to some degree at any time and is chronically at an increased risk for suicide. In some chronically suicidal patients with personality disorders, psychiatric hospitalization is used only as a last resort because the hospitalization is unlikely to change the chronic sui-cidal ideation. In fact, for such patients hospitalization may reinforce the sui-cidal ideation by creating an escape or gratifying a regressive need for attention. Short admissions, focused on stabilization and maintaining an out-patient treatment program, are usually most effective for the patient with a chronic high baseline risk for suicide. These complex patients require the active management that a mental health specialist can provide.

◼ Potentiating Risk Factors for Suicide

Exacerbation of depression with severe hopelessness, psychic pain, shame, or humiliation acutely increases risk of suicide. Depressive symptoms combined with extreme anxiety (e.g., panic or obsessions) or manic symptoms particularly increase risk (see Chapters 4 and 6). The initial treatment plan should target these exacerbated symptoms (see Treatment sections of Chapters 4 and 6). The risk of suicide seems highest in the first few depressive episodes, especially in late-onset depression. This is also true for bipolar disorders and schizophrenia. Many of the suicides that occur early in the course of the disorder are in people who have not been diagnosed with a disorder nor have initiated treatment. Though the risk of suicide is higher early in the course of an illness, the risk remains higher than in the general population throughout the course of the illness.

When psychosis is present, suicidal ideation is very dangerous and constitutes an emergency, particularly when command hallucinations or intense persecutory delusions are present (see Chapter 11 for further discussion on psychosis).

Extreme loss or abrupt social disruptions, such as divorce or the loss of a job, also increase acute risk. Following a spouse's death in later life is a particularly vulnerable period. The losses and disruptions of life posed by medical illness can be devastating.

Like psychiatric disorders, medical disorders pose acute and chronic risks. Much of the increased risk seen with medical disorders is attributable to co-occurring psychiatric illnesses, particularly major depression, substance-related disorders, personality disorders, and delirium. Physical illness is a profound risk factor, contributing to over 70% of suicides in those over the age of 60. Chronic medical illness is strongly associated with depression and substance abuse. However, even when the latter risk factors are accounted for, medical illness remains an independent risk factor for suicide. Higher rates of suicide have been reported in cancer, AIDS, end-stage renal disease, neurological disorders such as multiple sclerosis and asthma, and a number of other medical conditions. Data from the US National Comorbidity Survey (2) identified a dozen general medical diagnostic categories with significantly elevated odds ratios for suicide attempts, most ranging from 1.1 to 3.4, but with much higher odds ratios in AIDS, cancer, and asthma patients—each have a 4-fold risk of attempting suicide compared to the general population, even after adjusting for demographic and psychiatric variables. Poor or declining functional capacity and associated chronic pain may be a common thread among these medical conditions that links them with the risk of suicide. Some clinicians have the misperception that most terminally ill patients have a strong wish for a hastened death. On the contrary, Breitbart's 2000 study showed that only 17% of cancer patients had this desire; of those who desired a hastened death, the presence of depression was a strong predictor and not their diagnoses (3).

■ Protective Factors

The presence of protective factors can decrease risk, and their absence can increase risk, for suicide. Protective factors often involve the patient's relationships. Married people are at a lower risk than isolated people (e.g., those who are single, divorced, or widowed). Households with children under the age of 18 years seem to provide some protection for the adults in that household. Employment or meaningful work appears protective.

Increasing or augmenting protective factors is an important focus of treatment. In addition to pharmacotherapy for Ms A, a treatment plan that increases her contact with her grandchildren, maintains her attendance and functioning at work, and supports her connecting with others through her religious affiliation all decrease the overall risk for suicide; the risk, however, is never zero.

Religious affiliation may have some protective value above that of social contact in general. Studies of the relationship between religion and depression suggest that belief in a "higher power" is protective against depression in the elderly whether they practice collectively or independently. Though difficult to study, "a reason for living" has tremendous value clinically. Discussing protective factors takes time, but the information obtained focuses the management for both the patient and clinician.

■ Lethality of Suicide Plan

The risk of completed suicide also depends on the method contemplated by the patient, the extent of planning, and the patient's ability to access the means. The general rule follows: The more predictably lethal the contemplated method, the higher the risk. Patients who say they think about shooting themselves, hanging, inhaling carbon monoxide, or cutting their throats are usually at more risk than those who think about overdosing, cutting their wrists, stepping into traffic, or crashing their cars. Ironically, many who take potentially lethal overdoses of acetaminophen or aspirin do not realize how dangerous these overdoses are and did not truly intend to commit suicide.

Degree of planning is also important. A patient who has read up on the lethality of overdose options (information all too readily available on the Internet) and planned his or her attempt to take place when and where he or she will not be discovered by others is at a far greater risk than another patient who vaguely speaks of overdosing.

Finally, access to lethal means (e.g., firearms, dangerous prescription drugs such as insulin or barbiturates, and other toxins such as bromcoumarin or insecticides) raises the risk of suicide considerably.

■ Assessment and Management

As a clinician's interviewing and screening skills improve, he or she is likely to discover more suicidal ideation than previously anticipated; however, most patients with thoughts about suicide will not be at imminent risk for suicide nor will they require emergency interventions. The following steps guide the management of patients with suicidal ideation:

- Assess and compare the patient's current and baseline risks for suicide.
- Decide if there is imminent risk for suicide. (Is an attempt is likely in the next 24 to 48 hours?)
- Assess the support system available to the patient.
- Assess the lethality of the patient's suicide plan and means.
- Determine what setting is required for the initial steps of management.
- Make the management plan explicit with the patient, including follow-up and emergency contact.
- Document the assessment of suicidal risk and the plan.

■ Current Risk for Suicide vs Baseline Risk

Management of the patient experiencing suicidal ideation focuses on reducing the current risk to the baseline (and lower if possible). Several important points are critical:

- The risk is never zero.
- Some risks are not modifiable (i.e., gender, age, race, and past history).
- Some patients carry very high baseline risks for suicide.
- Some people will commit suicide despite a full assessment and good management.

Sudden change in risk is often more indicative of an imminent suicide attempt than the degree of risk alone and may not be associated with an increase in chronic risk. People with low baseline risks who suddenly have a major change (e.g., sudden illness, death of a loved one, or intoxication) may not have a sustained period of increased risk, but relative to their low baseline risks they have a major shift in risk and can be vulnerable to suicide. On the other hand, someone who carries a high baseline risk may actually have a higher absolute risk than the previous patient, but he or she may not be at any more imminent risk than they have been for years if no recent changes have occurred. Remember that while completed suicide is rare, suicide attempts, suicidal gestures, and ideation are common in psychiatric disorders. Clinicians cannot always prevent suicide, but they can assess and potentially reduce the risks for suicide attempts and completed suicides.

■ Imminent Risk for Suicide: Is an Attempt Likely in the Next 24 to 48 Hours?

Imminent risk is easy to determine when a patient has a clear plan for suicide and the intent to carry it out (or has just attempted suicide). Unpredictable patients (e.g., those who are psychotic or intoxicated) are also likely to have imminent risks because it is very hard to form a relationship with such a patient. There is no scale to weigh the many risk factors present against the protective factors or prohibitions against suicide that are also present. Clinical judgment is the only tool available to weigh the risks.

Assess the Support System Available to the Patient

Determining the patient's support system is a crucial component of fully assessing the patient's risk factors for suicide. If the patient is actively psychotic, has recently attempted suicide, or appears to be at high risk for suicide, then the hospital is the safest place for this patient. However, if the patient's symptoms permit outpatient treatment and the patient has an actively involved, well-functioning family that is capable and willing to be with the patient, then this patient potentially may be treated as an outpatient as long as there is no more than a moderate risk for suicide. This situation may also occur when a patient lives in a structured environment where observation is available. On the other hand, a patient with no social support may require hospitalization even if he or she has a lower level of risk. Such determinations are best made by mental health professionals. When an active support system is present, it is ideal to include that system in the management plan regardless of the setting for treatment.

What Setting Is Required for the Initial Steps of Management?

Closely related to assessing the support system is determining the setting for the next steps in the management plan. Practically speaking, there are usually just 2 options—home or the hospital. Legal and ethical principles require us to use the least restrictive setting while maintaining safety and effective management; this is often a difficult balancing act. Limitations in the availability of psychiatric hospitalization have shifted the treatment of psychiatric disorders toward the outpatient setting. Using support staff (i.e., social workers, nurses, or community services) can help form a support system for the at-risk patient. When the risk for suicide is imminent, inpatient hospitalization is required in a secure unit staffed with skilled professionals.

Make the Management Plan Explicit

Reviewing the details of the management plan with the patient helps actively enlist him or her in the treatment. Communicating the plan to the support system, when available, is also important for longitudinal management and decision making. When the patient refuses to involve his or her support system, the clinician is placed in a tough spot in regard to maintaining confidentiality (see section titled Confidentiality).

Though a "contract for safety" is used frequently, it is often overvalued and erroneously perceived as if it had the weight of a legal document. Contracts for safety, which are sometimes referred to as "no-harm contracts" or "suicide contracts," were originally conceived to facilitate the management of the suicidal patient. These contracts are vehicles used to articulate the treatment plan with parameters for increasing treatment intensity. The utility of this approach lies in both the explicit nature of the communication and the explicit agreement of the patient to the plan. The absence of the patient's agreement is an indication to consider psychiatric admission. Though contracts for safety can be a helpful communication tool, when used alone they provide little protective value for a patient who is intent on committing suicide.

Confidentiality

Patients who insist that "no one knows" about their depression, especially their suicidality, present a unique challenge. On one hand, confidentiality is a fundamental element of the clinician-patient relationship. On the other hand, maintaining safety for the patient may require a breach of that confidentiality. Generally, there is no need to break confidentiality if the patient does not have a high acute risk of suicide. However, confronting the secrecy of a patient who is creating isolation from significant support is appropriate. Asking the patient to call or bring a significant support person (e.g., spouse, family member, or friend) can be a fruitful intervention.

When significant suicidality is present and the clinician feels that there is an imminent suicide risk, then the clinician is required to act to ensure the safety of the patient. This includes breaking confidentiality and contacting others. As an alternative, the clinician may request that the patient contact his or her support system while he or she is still in the office with the clinician. This provides an opportunity to mobilize the patient's support system to closely attend to the patient and help ensure follow-through with a mental health referral when warranted.

■ Documentation

Legal liability is an important consideration in the management of suicidality. Patient suicides are the most frequent cause of legal action against psychiatrists. Any clinician who treats patients with mental disorders, especially depression, should document interactions carefully. The clinician should explicitly state the patient's risk factors and protective factors and describe the patient's support system, including who has been informed. The plan for continued care and the fact that the patient knows when and how to contact emergency services should be documented (see Box 2-4).

Box 2-4 Example of Documentation

Ms A comes in for a follow-up regarding her major depression and dysthymia. She says her symptoms of depression are not better, she appears more hopeless, and she expresses vague thoughts of suicide. Her current medication is 100 mg of sertraline each day for 8 weeks.

Target symptoms
Episodic suicidality; no suicide plan.
Prohibitions: grandchildren, work, and religion.
Initial insomnia and fatigue.
Hopelessness, isolation, and anhedonia are also present.
No access to guns.
No mania, psychosis, or anxiety present.

Assessment
Major depression in a patient with history of dysthymia, worsening symptoms. Suicidal ideation: vague, episodic with strong prohibitions. Patient's husband comes in and agrees with plan and feels she can be managed at home. Reviewed how to contact on-call clinicians and when to go to the ER.

Plan
Increase sertraline to 150 mg.
Add zolpidem 5 mg at bedtime.
Contact by telephone in 2 days for reassessment and return next week for follow-up. Patient and husband agree to plan as outlined above.

A good note facilitates patient care and communicates the plan to other providers. In addition, it helps protect the clinician in the event the patient completes suicide. The clinician's notes are the most reliable, and usually the only, records of treatment. Plaintiff's attorneys will assert that if you didn't write it, then you didn't do it. Remember, the goal is a complete assessment and appropriate management to address risk factors and maximize protective factors. Even when all is done correctly, however, some patients may still commit suicide.

The Use of Antidepressants and the Risk of Suicide

In the fall of 2004, the Food and Drug Administration (FDA) gave antidepressants as a class a "black box warning"—the most serious warning—stating: "Antidepressants increased the risk of suicidal thinking and behavior (suicidality) in short-term studies in children and adolescents with major depressive disorder (MDD) and other psychiatric disorders" (4,5). This warning was in part based on the pooled analysis of 24 trials and 4400 patients. They concluded that the risk of suicidality was 4% in patients receiving antidepressants and 2% in patients receiving placebo. *No suicides occurred in any of these trials.* The change in labeling was intended to motivate clinicians to discuss the potential for suicide, to explore risks factors associated with suicide, and to more closely monitor their patients. Instead, it generated many questions and confusion among clinicians and patients alike, and had the unintended effect of prompting patients (children, adolescents, and adults) to stop taking their antidepressants because of the misperception that antidepressants cause suicide.

In response, the FDA expanded its review of antidepressants and has ultimately published new recommendations and a medication guide regarding the use of antidepressants and suicidality (6) (see Appendix for the complete document). The FDA recommendations as of May 2007 are summarized below:

- Suicidal ideation and suicidality may increase during initial treatment with antidepressants in young adults 18 to 25 years old.
- The scientific data did *not* show this increased risk in adults older than 24 years nor in adults ages 65 and older.
- The future warning statements will emphasize that depression and certain other serious psychiatric disorders are themselves the most important causes of suicide (7).

It is our hope that these recommendations will have the original intended effect—to encourage clinicians to discuss the potential for suicide, to explore risks factors associated with suicide, and to more closely monitor their patients. The medication guide provided by the FDA is an excellent resource for both clinicians and patients alike.

When discussing the risk of suicidality, several key points should be emphasized with patients:

- Note that suicidal ideation may increase with initial treatment. (Current thinking suggests that this could be agitation or anxiety caused by the drug or the potential unmasking of latent bipolar disorder.)
- Tell the patient that the increased risk for suicidality is *not* associated with long-term use.
- Emphasize to the patient that he or she should *not* abruptly stop an antidepressant because abrupt cessation of medications is associated with significant side effects and risks, including increased suicidality.

KEY POINTS

- Suicidal thoughts and attempts are extremely common, but completed suicide is not.
- The clinical goal is to fully assess the risk for suicide, not predict it.

- Most suicides are the final event in a continuum that begins with negativity and hopelessness.
- Screening for suicide should begin with discussing hopelessness and negativity.
- If suicidal ideation is present, then fully assess risk factors:
  - Chronic/predisposing factors (e.g., gender, family history, age)
  - Acute/potentiating factors (e.g., recent loss of a loved one, exacerbation of an illness, access to firearms)
  - Protective factors (e.g., social support, children under the age of 18 in the home, religious beliefs)
  - Lethality of suicide plan
- Stratify suicide risk into imminent, acute, or chronic.
- Devise a plan addressing the risk factors and name the degree of risk.
- Fully document the plan in the medical record.

REFERENCES

1. Klonsky ED, Oltmanns TF, Turkheimer E. Deliberate self-harm in a nonclinical population: Prevalence and psychological correlates. *Am J Psychiatry.* 2003;160:1501-1508.

2. Goodwin R, Marusic A, Hoven C. Suicide attempts in the United States: The role of physical illness. *Soc Sci Med.* 2003; 56:1783-1788.

3. Breitbart W, Rosenfeld B, Pessin H, et al. Depression, hopelessness, and desire for hastened death in terminally ill patients with cancer. *JAMA.* 2000;284:2907-2911.

4. US Food and Drug Administration. Labeling change request letter for antidepressant medications. Available at: http://www.fda.gov/cder/drug/antidepressants/SSRIlabelChange.htm. Accessed August 17, 2007.

5. US Food and Drug Administration. FDA public health advisory: Suicidality in adults being treated with antidepressant medications. Available at: http://www.fda.gov/CDER/DRUG/advisory/SSRI200507.htm. Accessed August 17, 2007.

6. US Food and Drug Administration. Medication guide: antidepressant medicines, depression and other serious mental illnesses, and suicidal thoughts or actions. Available at: http://www.fda.gov/cder/drug/antidepressants/antidepressants_MG_2007.pdf. Accessed August 17, 2007.

7. US Food and Drug Administration. FDA proposes new warnings about suicidal thinking, behavior in young adults who take antidepressant medications. Available at: http://www.fda.gov/bbs/topics/NEWS/2007/NEW01624.html. Accessed August 17, 2007.

KEY REFERENCES

American Psychiatric Association's practice guideline for the assessment and treatment of patients with suicidal behaviors. *Am J Psychiatry.* 2003;160.

Block SD. Assessing and managing depression in the terminally ill patient. *Ann Intern Med.* 2000;132:209-218.

Bostwick JM, Levenson JL. Suicidality. In: Levenson JL, ed. *American Psychiatric Publishing Textbook of Psychosomatic Medicine*. Washington, DC: American Psychiatric Publishing, Inc; 2005:219-234.

Copsey Spring TR, Yanni LM, Levenson JL. A shot in the dark: Failing to recognize the link between physical and mental illness. *J Gen Intern Med* (in press).

Harris EC, Barraclough BM. Suicide as an outcome for medical disorders. *Medicine*. 1994;73:281-389.

Khan A, Khan S, Kolts R, Brown WA. Suicide rates in clinical trials of SSRIs, other antidepressants, and placebo: Analysis of FDA reports. *Am J Psychiatry*. 2003; 169:790-792.

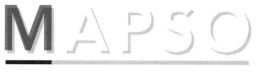

MAPSO

Mood
Disorders

Depression: Evaluation and Case-Finding Strategies

■ Depression and the Role of the General Clinician in Its Evaluation and Diagnosis

The general clinician is confronted daily with patients who have some component of depression. The clinician's complex task is to first recognize when some sign of depression is present and then determine if the mood disturbance is an isolated symptom or part of a group of symptoms that constitute a disorder. Mood disorders are the group of disorders in the DSM-IV that have a mood disturbance (e.g., depression) as the central symptom. Major depression is the most common mood disorder and is the most common mental disorder seen in the primary care setting. In fact, it is the second most common disorder seen, second only to hypertension. Yet often it is not recognized and, when recognized, it is not properly treated. Also, the diagnosis of "depression" is frequently incorrectly assigned to another psychiatric disorder (e.g., alcohol dependence), a "normal" condition (e.g., bereavement), or a medical disorder (e.g., sleep apnea). The purpose of this chapter is to provide the necessary terms, concepts, and case-finding strategies required by the general clinician to correctly recognize and diagnose mood disorders (e.g., major depression) in the primary care setting.

Essential Concepts and Terms

The confusing terminology used to describe mood disorders and depression significantly contributes to underrecognition and incorrect treatment of mood disorders. The word "depression" is nonspecific; it can signify a normal emotion, an abnormal symptom, or a set of clinical syndromes. Also, the words "affective," "mood," and "depressive" are used interchangeably. Knowing and understanding the terminology is essential to recognition and accurate diagnostic formulation. To use and understand evidence-based treatments, the clinician has to be fluent in the terminology and concepts used in the studies.

Major Depression

The DSM-IV describes major depression as a clinical syndrome (i.e., disorder) characterized by a total of at least 5 symptoms, including a depressed mood or anhedonia, every day, all day for at least 2 weeks with significant functional impairment (see Box 3-1). About 1 in 10 primary care adult out-patients have major depression or dysthymia. Although major depression can occur at any age, the disorder often first develops between the ages of 25 and 44. The lifetime prevalence of depression in community samples varies between 10% and 24% for women and between 5% and 12% for men.

Box 3-1 Major Depression: DSM-IV Criteria

1. Depressed mood and/or anhedonia every day, all day for at least 2 weeks
2. At least 4 additional symptoms (i.e., 5 or more total symptoms)
   a. Neurovegetative symptoms
      i. Sleep changes
      ii. Fatigue
      iii. Appetite or weight changes
      iv. Psychomotor retardation or agitation
      v. Difficulty concentrating or making decisions
   b. Psychological symptoms
      i. Helplessness
      ii. Hopelessness (e.g., excessive guilt)
      iii. Frequent thoughts of death or suicide
3. Significant impairment in functioning

Major depression is frequently accompanied by other psychiatric disorders. For example, the National Comorbidity Study Replication (NCS-R) found that most lifetime (72.1%) and 12-month (78.5%) cases had comorbid DSM-IV disorders (1).

When clinicians screen for a depressed mood as a symptom, they often fail to check for the additional symptoms and functional impairment required when establishing the diagnosis of major depression. Their fore-shortened approach can lead to misdiagnosing "normal-range" depressed mood as major depression, missing the diagnosis of a different mood disorder (e.g., dysthymia or a bipolar disorder), or failing to detect another disorder (e.g., anxiety disorder) when present. We use the term "symptom density" to emphasize the point that the greater the number (i.e., "density") of symptoms a patient has, the greater the likelihood that one or more disorders are present that will benefit from treatment.

Dysthymia

Dysthymia, another mood disorder, is characterized by a depressed mood *or* anhedonia plus at least 2 additional symptoms (i.e., a total of 3 symptoms) of depression for 2 or more years (see Box 3-2). Dysthymia affects 3% to 6% of individuals in the community and carries the same risk for disability as major depression. It is frequently comorbid with other psychiatric disorders. Co-occurring dysthymia with an episode of major depression is referred to as "double depression." Double depression is more difficult to treat, and relapse is more likely than with either disorder alone. Given dysthymia's chronicity, many patients fail to attribute the depressive symptoms to a disorder but rather ascribe the symptoms to their character. The patient may say, "I am just a depressed-type person." This perception represents an integration of depressive symptoms into the person's character and may make dysthymia harder to diagnosis and treat because the patient may not view the symptoms as "abnormal" for himself or herself.

Box 3-2 Dysthymia: DSM-IV Criteria

---

1. Depressed mood or anhedonia
2. At least 2 additional symptoms:
   a. Appetite changes
   b. Sleep changes
   c. Fatigue, low energy
   d. Hopelessness
   e. Poor self-esteem
   f. Poor concentration, difficulty with decision making
3. Symptoms all present for 2 or more years
4. Symptoms never abate for more than 2 months
5. No episode of major depression during the 2-year period or for 6 months prior to symptom onset

---

■ Case-Finding Strategies

Screening for Depression and the Likelihood of False Positives

When a major depressive disorder is suspected, the simplest sensitive screening question is, *Are you feeling depressed, sad, or blue?* This single question is 90% sensitive in detecting major depressive disorders, but its specificity is only 57% (Table 3-1). If an additional question looking for anhedonia is added (*Have you lost interest in, or do you have a decreased desire to do, things that used to be pleasurable?*), then the screening questions' sensitivity increases to 95%, and the specificity increases to 90% (Table 3-2). The real impact of the additional question and subsequent increase in sensitivity and specificity plays out in the reduction in the number of false-positive responses from 40 false-positive responses with the one-question screening strategy to 9 false-positive responses with the two-question screening strategy. In other words, the clinician will identify over 5 times as many "depressed" patients (40 vs 7) without major depression as compared to "depressed" patients with a major mood disorder.

The false positives represent a group of people with nonpsychiatric disorders (i.e., medical mimics), subsyndromal (i.e., mild) depressive disorders, other psychiatric disorders (e.g., anxiety disorders), or "normal" depressive feelings in reaction to a stressor (i.e., grief). These "false positives" do not have major depression, but they are a focus of clinical interest in their own right because, when they are followed over time, they have greater functional impairment and higher rates of recent use of mental health services.

Table 3-1 One Screening Question, "Are you depressed?"

100 patients screened	Major mood disorder present	No major mood disorder present
47 (Test positive) "Yes, I am depressed"	7 (True positive)	40 (False positive)
53 (Test negative) "No, I don't feel depressed"	1 (False negative)	52 (True negative)

Assume 8% prevalence of major depression or dysthymia,
"Do you feel depressed?": 90% sensitivity, and 57% specificity

Table 3-2 Two Screening Questions, "Are you depressed?" and "Have you lost interest in things?"

100 patients screened	Major mood disorder present	No major mood disorder present
17 (Test positive) "Yes" to both	8 (True positive)	9 (False positive)
83 (Test negative) "No" to either one or both	0 (False negative)	83 (True negative)

Assume 8% prevalence of major depression or dysthymia.
"Do you feel depressed?" and "Have you lost interest in doing things?": 95% sensitivity and 90% specificity

Should We Screen All Patients for Depression?

The US Preventive Services Task Force (USPSTF) recommended screening *all* adults for depression in clinical practices *if* health care delivery systems are in place to assure accurate diagnosis, effective treatment, and follow-up (2). However, health care delivery systems that assure accurate diagnosis, effective treatment, and follow-up are difficult to define in general medical practices and are probably rare. Screening *all* patients (including those not reporting depressive symptoms) for depression is time consuming for practitioners, so some practices have instituted self-administered screening instruments that patients can fill out in the waiting room. This approach is very sensitive, but to gain the required specificity, a skilled clinician must subsequently ask follow-up questions during the patient's exam.

The USPSTF links its screening recommendation to practices in which a well-functioning treatment system is in place for major depressive disorders. An effective treatment system has typically meant a general clinician's office that supports accurate diagnosis, prescription of effective treatments, careful follow-up, and access to a specialty mental health system. These are significant preconditions for screening *all* patients. Many clinicians do not conduct unselected screening efforts, instead utilizing case-finding strategies only when an index of suspicion is raised (i.e., when the patient has depressive symptoms or a past history of a major mood disorder or in a population of patients in which the incidence of depression is very high). This selective-screening approach decreases the number of false positives and raises the number of true positives as noted previously. This latter approach is probably most typical, but it fails to address the USPSTF's recommendation of having an effective system for complete care. The bare minimum of such a system is a capable and willing general clinician who has both emergency contact phone numbers (i.e., "crisis lines") and community mental health contacts.

■ Considering Medical Mimics

Medical conditions and substances, both abused and therapeutic, are frequently associated with abnormal mood symptoms and should be considered early in the clinical process when a psychiatric diagnosis is suspected (see Box 3-3). Endocrinopathies, malignancies, chronic infectious diseases, and cerebrovascular disease are all major medical conditions that can cause mood symptoms. Substance-induced mood disorders include not only substances of abuse (e.g., alcohol, cocaine) but also prescription medications (e.g., corticosteroids), over-the-counter medications (e.g., pseudoephedrine), and substances not typically associated with abuse (e.g., caffeine).

> **Box 3-3 Selected Medical Mimics with Mood Symptoms**
>
> 1. Endocrinopathies (e.g., hypothyroidism and hyperthyroidism, hypoadrenalism and hyperadrenalism)
> 2. Pancreatic cancer
> 3. Chronic viral infections (e.g., HIV, hepatitis C, cytomegalovirus [CMV], Epstein-Barr virus [EBV])
> 4. Stroke
> 5. Neurological diseases (e.g., Parkinson disease, multiple sclerosis)
> 6. Substances of abuse (e.g., alcohol, cocaine, amphetamines)
> 7. Psychoactive substances (e.g., caffeine, OTC sympathomimetics)
> 8. Medications (e.g., corticosteroids, hormonal therapies, interferons, anticancer agents, older antihypertensives)

Alcohol is one of the most common mood-altering substances in this category. In this instance, the task is to distinguish between dual diagnoses (e.g., depression plus alcoholism) or a purely alcohol-induced mood disturbance. Though the acute effects of alcohol may be gone in less than 24 hours, the chronic and often depressive effects may linger for 6 to 12 weeks if alcohol is heavily ingested daily. Because many alcoholic patients minimize or deny alcohol use, a high index of suspicion is required in the evaluation of a patient with depressive symptoms not otherwise accounted for.

Other substances, including cocaine and amphetamines, can create an intense depressive state during withdrawal, whereas chronic marijuana use can create a subtle state of depression with lack of motivation and decreased emotional reactivity. Substance use does not have to be excessive to alter mood. Some people are vulnerable to the depressive effects of these substances even with moderate use. *Substance-induced mood disorders should be especially considered when patients are not responding to treatment.*

Detailed discussions of psychoactive substances, including medications, are found in Chapter 12. Several examples of commonly prescribed medications are briefly mentioned in this section. The list of agents that can cause depressive symptoms is long, but corticosteroids and interferons are among the most commonly used agents that cause depressive symptoms. Common psychoactive substances like caffeine are often overlooked when considering depression. Excessive use of caffeine can cause anxiety, irritability, and insomnia. The caffeine-induced insomnia results in fatigue, which leads to an increase in caffeine consumption, thus perpetuating the cycle of caffeine use. Caffeine withdrawal can result in intermittent depressed mood, irritability, fatigue, headache, and decreased concentration—mimicking minor depression.

■ Differentiating Subsyndromal Depressive Symptoms from Major Depressive and Dysthymic Disorders

Subsyndromal Depression

Minor depression, or subsyndromal depression, has depressed mood as its core symptom. However, it lacks the severity of major depression or the chronicity of dysthymia. The DSM-IV considers it a provisional diagnosis requiring further investigation. Its purpose for discussion here lies in its value, conceptually, as a subsyndromal state and its impact on functioning when it persists for 2 years (i.e., dysthymia) or when it represents a prodromal state of major depression. Minor depression is defined as a depressed mood and 2 additional symptoms (never more than 5 symptoms total) lasting at least 2 weeks.

Minor depression tends to resolve spontaneously—irrespective of treatment—in 3 months or less. However, minor or subsyndromal depression is a strong risk factor for major depression. This appears to be particularly true in late-onset depression. A clinical approach that includes reassurance, encouragement, supportive listening, problem solving, and community involvement is probably the best way to manage these patients over time. The evidence regarding treatment of minor depression is evolving, but the current focus of treatment is either on the dominant symptom (i.e., target symptom) that is causing the most distress or on the stressor precipitating the symptoms, not on long-term antidepressant treatment. Rather, antidepressant therapy should be reserved for major depressive disorders because antidepressants often require 90 days to reach full effectiveness and then should be continued for at least 6 more months. As previously noted, many of the episodes of minor depression resolve without treatment. A major risk of antidepressant therapy in minor depression is that the clinician and patient could misinterpret the resolution of symptoms as a beneficial response to treatment.

A broad range of interventions, including pharmacologic, psychotherapeutic, behavioral, social, and lifestyle interventions, are used in the management of symptoms of subsyndromal depressive disorders. The patient's preference is the primary consideration in choosing the intervention. The symptomatic management of mood symptoms is discussed in detail at the end of Chapter 4.

■ Bereavement and Grief

Individual expression of grief during bereavement varies considerably. Culture, religion, and personal experiences greatly influence the experience. It is hard to predict which losses will impact individuals most. Some losses will hurt far more and take longer to resolve than others; losses that may seem minor to others are nevertheless profound for the patient (e.g., loss of pet). Depressive symptoms are common and often intense during periods of bereavement but do not require treatment with antidepressant medication unless major depression is also present. Bereavement may cause suffering, but it is not an illness or disorder. It seems counterintuitive to some that "suffering" could be a normal and healthy response for some situations.

The clinical dilemma when assessing a grieving patient is whether or not a psychiatric disorder (usually major depression) is also present and whether or not the patient would benefit from treatment. Antidepressants tend to be overprescribed to grieving patients, but only those who meet criteria for depression should receive them. Instead, agents that target specific symptoms (e.g., sedative hypnotics) and psychotherapy may be helpful in some cases. Interestingly, current evidence suggests that treatment of major depression during bereavement decreases the symptoms of major depression but does not affect the grief. Some grief reactions, especially when the relationship with the deceased was complex and conflicted, can become chronic and persistent; this situation usually indicates a need for a referral for psychotherapy, as opposed to medications.

"Normal" or typical bereavement manifests differently from major depression across several important domains (see Table 3-3). Bereavement

Table 3-3 Comparison of Bereavement and Major Depression

Symptom	Bereavement	Major Depression
Suicidality	Absent	Present
Psychosis	Absent	Present
Affect	Some positive	Mostly depressed
Degree of dysfunction	Mild to moderate	Severe
Guilt	Mild	May be severe
Self-perception	Normal	Unwell
Psychomotor retardation	Absent	Present
Sleeplessness	Present	Present
Duration	Usually less than 2 months	Longer and worsening symptoms
History of depressive illness	No personal or family history	Personal or family history often present

tends to be shorter in duration, is not viewed as a disorder by the bereaved, and results in only minor impairment of functioning. Frequently, the depressive symptoms are less severe and not as persistent. In bereavement, a patient's depressed affect is intermittently present, whereas in major depression, the affect is usually pervasively depressed with little variation. Typically, bereavement does not worsen over time, but rather gradually lessens in intensity. It is not known why some bereaving people have hallucinations, but auditory and visual hallucinations may occur in normal bereavement. Unlike the hallucinations in psychotic depression, the hallucinations in bereavement are typically reassuring, brief, and limited to the voice or image of the deceased. In psychotic depression, the hallucinations are troubling, more pervasive, and can correspond to various voices, sounds, and images.

Management of bereavement starts with ruling out a major psychiatric disorder. Carefully reviewing past symptoms provides valuable information for comparison with the current symptoms. Patients with a past history of major depression or another psychiatric illness are at risk for a recurrence or exacerbation of their disorder during bereavement. When major psychopathology is not found or is unclear, then symptomatic management and supportive, attentive follow-up is indicated. This approach is very similar to that used in minor depression. Sleeplessness is extremely common, and the use of a sedative-hypnotic may be very helpful. Targeting one or more symptoms that are most distressing should guide treatment. It is also appropriate to explore how the grief is processed. Support from religious affiliations, support groups, friends, and family may all be helpful. A professional therapist may also help the patient understand and cope during more complicated bereavement reactions. In any case, a full assessment combined with the clinician's tolerance for his or her own grief is critical. In other words, if clinicians have difficulty handling their grief personally, then they will have difficulty handling patients' grief reactions, too.

Case Study

Mr Z is a 67-year-old man who comes in for his blood pressure checkup. He appears lethargic, and his blood pressure is 190/90. He reports that his older brother died 3 weeks ago and he's "not doing so good with it." He notes that he sleeps poorly, has been tearful when going through his brother's belongings with his brother's wife, and has not wanted to do much. He has been able to continue working full time. He has no suicidal thoughts but does think about his own death. He has no past history of depression. He may be drinking more alcohol than previously. He has no past history of alcohol abuse, and his intake is 2 drinks per night to "help him sleep." Mr Z is tearful when discussing his brother, but he regains his composure in just a few minutes.

Mr Z's symptoms fall well within normal boundaries of bereavement. Though very symptomatic, he is able to circumscribe his feelings and continue to function well. An antidepressant would probably not relieve his symptoms because he does not have major depression. Instead, an approach that includes validating his grief, reducing his alcohol intake, and providing an alternative for sleeplessness are appropriate. Close follow-up to watch for worsening symptoms or increasing alcohol consumption completes the plan.

■ Seasonal Affective Disorder

Seasonal affective disorder (SAD) is a mood disorder consisting of recurrent episodes of major depression that occur with a seasonal pattern, most commonly with depressive episodes during the fall and winter and full remission to normal mood (or switching to hypomania or mania) during the spring and summer. Randomized controlled trials with light therapy have demonstrated short-term improvement in SAD, but little is known regarding light therapy's long-term benefits. A variety of modalities have been tested, including light boxes, light visors, and dawn simulators. The therapeutic effects are mediated via the eyes, not the skin. The intensity of the light—on the order of 10,000 lux—is probably a requirement to achieve benefits. The ideal timing remains controversial, but most controlled trials have shown morning light to be superior to evening light. The optimal dose has not been determined. Side effects include minor visual complaints, headache, insomnia, and overactivation (rarely including mania). Most light therapy modalities screen out UV rays, so adverse cutaneous reactions are limited to patients with photosensitivity. There have been no reports of basal cell cancer or cataracts with light therapy. No ocular changes have been detected even after years of treatment, and there are no defined ocular contraindications. There is no evidence of similar benefits from tanning salons because eyes are usually covered and high UV light exposure carries risks. There is no evidence that replacing home or office light bulbs with bulbs of different spectra provides any benefit. There is some evidence of modest acute benefits of light therapy in nonseasonal depression but no evidence that it can be used instead of standard therapies. Even with SAD, light therapy is not adequate as the sole treatment if symptoms are severe.

◼ Screening for Bipolar Disorders and Psychosis

Establishing a diagnosis of a major mood disorder should include additional steps of screening for a history of mania, hypomania, and psychosis. Mania or hypomania are typically not present when a patient presents with a depressive episode, but either may have been present previously. The exception is a mixed episode in bipolar disorder (see Chapter 6). It is important to rule out bipolar disorder before initiating treatment because the treatments for major depression (i.e., unipolar depression) and bipolar depression are different. In fact, treating the depressive phase of a bipolar disorder with an antidepressant alone (i.e., without a mood stabilizer present) runs the risk of "switching" or "flipping" the patient's depressive episode into a manic or hypomanic episode. Typically, a mood stabilizer is initiated before or sometimes in conjunction with an antidepressant when treating bipolar depression (see Chapter 6 for screening questions and information on treatment).

Psychosis can occur in up to 15% of major depressive episodes. The presence of psychotic symptoms is referred to as "psychotic depression" or "depression with psychotic features," and it often, but does not always, suggests that the patient has bipolar disorder. The most common psychotic symptoms experienced during a depressive episode are auditory hallucinations. Clinicians have incorrectly assumed that psychotic symptoms only occur in the most severe depressive episodes; in fact, psychotic symptoms can be present in moderate depression, too. However, detecting such symptoms requires active screening strategies (see Chapter 12).

■ Screening for Comorbidities

Medical and other psychiatric disorders frequently co-occur with depression. As noted previously, about 75% of patients with major depression experience a comorbid psychiatric disorder during their lives. The lifetime comorbidity with any anxiety disorder or substance use is 59% and 24%, respectively. Actively screening for the second diagnosis is critical because the presence of a comorbid disorder significantly affects treatment choices.

KEY POINTS

- The word "depression" is nonspecific and can refer to a normal emotion, an abnormal symptom, or a set of clinical syndromes.
- *Are you feeling sad or depressed?* is a 90% sensitive screening question for major mood disorders.
- Many false positives arise when entire populations (including asymptomatic people) are screened.
- If mental health resources are limited, then targeting screening to patients who are either exhibiting depressive symptoms or at high risk for a major mood disorder (e.g., personal history of depression, family history of depression) is recommended.
- First consider the possibility that the symptoms are caused by a medical condition or induced by a substance, including a medication.
- Minor depression, or subsyndromal depression, often resolves without treatment but may represent the beginning of a major depressive episode.
- Frequently, people who are grieving feel "depressed," but they usually do not have major depression that requires treatment.

REFERENCES

1. Kessler RC, Berglund P, Demler O, et al. Lifetime prevalence and age-of-onset distributions of DSM-IV disorders in the national comorbidity survey replication. *Arch Gen Psychiatry.* 2005;62:593-602.
2. USPSTF. Screening for depression: Recommendations from the US Preventive Services Task Force. *Ann Intern Med.* 2002;136:760-764.

KEY REFERENCES

Golden RN, Gaynes BN, Ekstrom RD, et al. The efficacy of light therapy in the treatment of mood disorders: A review and meta-analysis of the evidence. *Am J Psychiatry.* 2005;162:656-662.

Hensley PL. Treatment of bereavement-related depression and traumatic grief. *J Affect Disord.* 2006;92(1):117-124.

Kroenke K. Minor depression: midway between major depression and euthymia. *Ann Intern Med.* 2006;144:496-504.

Leon AC, Portera L, Olfson M, et al. False positive results: a challenge for psychiatric screening in primary care. *Am J Psychiatry.* 1997;15:1462-1464.

Magnusson A, Partonen T. The diagnosis, symptomatology, and epidemiology of seasonal affective disorder. *CNS Spectr.* 2005;10(8):625-634.

Rodin GM, Nolan RP, Katz MR. Depression. In: Levenson JL, ed. *American Psychiatric Publishing Textbook of Psychosomatic Medicine.* Washington DC: American Psychiatric Publishing, Inc; 2005:193-218.

Schneider RK, Glenn RN, Levenson JL. Chapter 4. In: Levenson JL, ed. *Depression.* Philadelphia: American College of Physicians; 2000: 76-96.

Whooley MA, Avins AL, Miranda J, Browner WS. Case-finding instruments for depression, two questions are as good as many. *J Gen Intern Med.* 1997;12:439-445.

Winkler D, Pjrek E, Iwaki R, Kasper S. Treatment of seasonal affective disorder. *Expert Rev Neurother.* 2006;6(7):1039-1048.

Zisook S, Shuchter SR, Sledge PA, et al. The spectrum of depressive phenomena after spousal bereavement. *J Clin Psychiatry.* 1994;55:29-36.

M

Treatment of Major Depression and Dysthymia: Initial Interventions

■ Treatment of Major Depression and Dysthymia and the Role of the General Clinician

About 1 in 10 primary care adult outpatients have major depression or dysthymia. Despite the high prevalence of major depressive disorders (MDD), the rates of detection and adequate treatment remain low. In one primary care survey, 52% of 12-month cases received health care treatment for MDD, and treatment was adequate in only 42% of these cases (1). Appropriate and effective treatment requires a complete pretreatment evaluation carefully establishing the diagnosis, characterizing the longitudinal course, identifying target symptoms, as well as assessing for suicidality (Chapter 2), possible bipolar illness (Chapter 6), psychosis (Chapter 12), and comorbid conditions.

■ General Strategies for Initial Treatment

The initial treatments for major depression and dysthymia fall into 2 major categories: psychotherapy and psychopharmacology (i.e., medications). Nonpsychotherapy and nonpsychopharmacology interventions such as exercise, diet, and religion are used only adjunctively in major depression and dysthymia or for the management of minor (i.e., subsyndromal) depression. Nonpharmacologic treatments are discussed at the end of this chapter.

The possible combinations of psychotherapy and medication create 4 initial outpatient treatment modalities for depression: (1) psychotherapy; (2) an antidepressant; (3) an antidepressant with an additional agent; or (4) psychotherapy in combination with one or more medications. One can expect a response rate between 40% and 60% with one of these initial treatment strategies, depending upon factors including the disorder (i.e., major depression vs dysthymia), the severity, the length of time for the response, and the comorbid conditions (both medical and psychiatric).

Pretreatment Considerations

When antidepressants are prescribed, most are only taken for 90 days or less. Misdiagnosis, overprescribing, and inadequate patient preparation contribute to this phenomenon. Treatments for depression are often initiated without sufficient pretreatment evaluation and education of the patient. Routinely reviewing key considerations prior to initiating treatment increases the chances for adherence and an optimal outcome for the patient. Key considerations are shown in Box 4-1.

Chapters 2 and 3 review key early steps when assessing a patient with depressive symptoms. These steps focus on ruling out other possible causes for the patient's depressive symptoms (e.g., medical mimics and subsyndromal disorders) and assessing the severity of the symptoms and the patient's safety. At this point, the clinician *can* establish a diagnosis *if* there are sufficient symptoms (i.e., if there is "symptom density") of sufficient severity and DSM-IV criteria for the disorder are met. It is important to remember that the diagnosis of any psychiatric disorder is ultimately a clinical judgment, not the product of a checklist (see Chapter 1).

> **Box 4-1 Key Considerations Prior to Initiating Treatment**
>
> 1. Rule out medical mimics and subsyndromal disorders (Chapter 3).
> 2. Establish the primary diagnosis.
> 3. Characterize the longitudinal course of symptoms.
> 4. Assess the spectrum of suicidality (Chapter 2).
> 5. Assess for a history of mania or hypomania (Chapter 6).
> 6. Assess for psychosis (Chapter 12).
> 7. Assess for comorbid conditions (e.g., medical, psychiatric, or substance abuse).
> 8. Identify the "target" symptoms (see Identifying Target Symptoms)
> 9. Determine patient preferences and past treatment outcomes and then establish reasonable expectations for the response to treatment.

Characterizing the Longitudinal Course of Depression

After detecting the presence of a major depressive episode, the *longitudinal course* is then characterized (i.e., single episode, recurrent episode, chronic depression, dysthymia, and recurrent depression plus dysthymia). Determining if (and how many) previous episodes have occurred and what the responses (or lack of responses) have been to prior treatments provides valuable information to guide current treatment and predict prognosis. While the current episode may be the first episode treated, a careful history may reveal past episodes that resolved without treatment. For example, the patient may indicate that "this time it has not gone away, and it is even worse." Generally, the longer symptoms have been present, the longer it can take to show a response to treatment.

The differences between the definitions of response, remission, and return to full functioning (i.e., recovery) are subtle but significant. *Response*

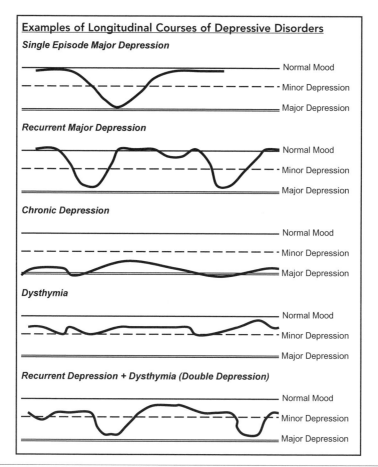

Examples of Longitudinal Courses of Depressive Disorders

Single Episode Major Depression

— Normal Mood
— Minor Depression
— Major Depression

Recurrent Major Depression

— Normal Mood
— Minor Depression
— Major Depression

Chronic Depression

— Normal Mood
— Minor Depression
— Major Depression

Dysthymia

— Normal Mood
— Minor Depression
— Major Depression

Recurrent Depression + Dysthymia (Double Depression)

— Normal Mood
— Minor Depression
— Major Depression

Figure 4-1

means either a 50% reduction in initial symptoms or a decrease in symptoms such that criteria for the disorder are no longer met. *Remission* means the resolution of all signs and symptoms of the disorder. In essence, remission means the absence of disorder-related symptoms. Typically, response rates are higher than remission rates. Though return to "normal functioning" is seldom measured in studies, it is certainly anticipated by our patients. *Recovery* refers to a prolonged state of remission.

Identifying Target Symptoms

Before initiating treatment, it is advisable to determine, then record, the patient's most troubling symptoms, which the treatment is "targeted" to relieve. Target symptoms are ideally quantifiable (e.g., sleep and weight changes, crying spells, inactivity, poor work attendance) and better than less specific markers like "feeling better." Target symptoms typically are associated with a significant and specific area of dysfunction. For example, irritability may be impacting the patient's relationship with his or her children; fatigue and poor concentration may be linked to poor work attendance or performance. A patient receiving treatment for major depression often does not "feel" better early on (and may not for many weeks) but may still have had a marked improvement with the target symptoms. This occurs because the patient's depressed mood is frequently one of the last symptoms to resolve in the treatment of depression. The patient who is having an early favorable response to treatment for depression may honestly respond, "I'm not feeling any better," but still have improvements in sleep, appetite, and energy. Often people other than the patient see improvement before the patient "feels" better. Noting the patient's target symptoms at the initiation of treatment gives the clinician and the patient valuable benchmarks to measure treatment response in the absence of "feeling better" and helps prevent premature changes (i.e., switching agents) or discontinuation of medication that may ultimately work very well.

Noting Patient Preferences and Past Treatment Outcomes

We are fortunate to live during a time when many effective treatments exist for major depression. Often patients have direct experience from prior treatment or information from other sources (e.g., family, friends, media) regarding treatments for depression. Unfortunately, some patients come in with information that is distorted or patently false. Sifting through what patients know gives the clinician a chance to reinforce the correct information and clarify mistakes and misunderstandings while determining the patient's preferences.

Rather than complying with a patient's wishes, engaging the patient's preferences sets the stage for dialogue and ultimately an alliance between the patient and the clinician. This alliance is integral to compliance and a favorable response. For example, a patient may assume a previously used antidepressant was ineffective and not want to take it. However, noting that the previous dosage was too low and treatment was too brief to expect positive results may allow the clinician to prescribe this potentially effective agent that previously "failed." Further discussion could explain that antidepressants require at least 6 to 12 weeks to take effect and dosages need to be increased to the maximum level tolerated. The alliance and dialogue build reasonable expectations that ultimately influence adherence and compliance. Introducing the idea of psychotherapy early in the process facilitates its acceptance and ultimately its effectiveness in managing acute and long-standing depressive symptoms. Also, exploring the utility of psychotherapy with patients helps shift away from the concept that medications "fix" everything and are the complete or easy answer.

Follow-Up and Duration of Treatment

According to current guidelines, clinicians should follow up every 1 to 2 weeks with patients being treated for depression until an adequate response occurs. For many busy clinicians and patients, frequent face-to-face visits are difficult and impractical. In these instances, a nurse's office visit or phone call may suffice. Patients have better adherence and responses to treatment, and fewer of them stop treatment if they have a closer follow-up (i.e., greater frequency of visits or clinician contacts).

There are depression scales that can be used (e.g., Beck Depression Inventory) to follow patients' responses to treatment. Tracking selected target symptoms (see Identifying Target Symptoms in this chapter) is a proxy for these more inclusive instruments. Tangible measures serve as a good guide for determining if further changes (e.g., increases) in medications are warranted. They provide data for the clinician and patient to discuss and utilize when making decisions to modify the treatment. When self-administered instruments are completed by patients while waiting for the clinician, the visit with the clinician can start with this valuable information. This is similar to efficient practices that have the patient's blood pressure or blood glucose measurements taken prior to the patient and clinician meeting face-to-face.

Treatment is divided into 3 phases: acute, continuation, and maintenance phases. The goal of the acute phase is remission; the goal of the continuation phase is to prevent a relapse of the current episode of depression; and the goal of the maintenance phase is to prevent the recurrence of a new episode. Length of treatment for a single episode is dictated by the time it takes for the symptoms to remit plus the time needed for continued

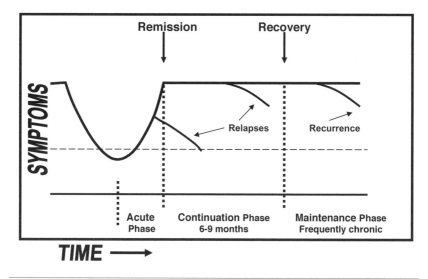

Figure 4-2

treatment to prevent a relapse. Continued long-term treatment (i.e., maintenance therapy) is recommended for those patients at high risk for recurrence of depression (e.g., those with multiple previous episodes, residual symptoms, chronic stressors, or comorbid diseases).

Acute Phase

The acute phase is *not* time dependent; the acute phase takes as long as it takes for symptoms to remit (i.e., remission). Acute-phase treatment begins with the initiation of treatment and ends when the patient has fully remitted and has no active symptoms. Most antidepressants have an onset of action in 2 to 4 weeks, and the maximum response for a given dose is reached by 6 to 12 weeks. However, many patients do not remit within 3 months and may require augmentation or a switch of antidepressants. The important point to remember is that the focus of acute-phase treatment is symptom remission and not the length of treatment; there is no "clock" per se in acute-phase treatment.

Continuation Phase

How long should antidepressant therapy be continued? The continuation phase is time dependent. Current recommendations suggest that the continuation phase should last 6 to 9 months after the first episode of depression has remitted. Depending on the population, the relapse rate without continuation therapy is about 50%, with most relapses occurring within 6 months after cessation of the medication. It is very important for patients to understand the need for continuation therapy. For a single episode of depression, the shortest duration of treatment possible—acute plus continuation phases—is 9 to 12 months.

Maintenance Phase and Prevention of Recurrence

The decision to continue treatment into the maintenance phase or to discontinue active treatment is a complex one and is ideally a joint doctor-patient decision made after weighing all the information. The most important considerations are the risk of recurrence, the severity of the depressive episodes, the side effects of treatment, and patient preference.

The risk of recurrence goes up with each successive depressive episode. The recurrence rate after 1 episode is 50% to 85%. Residual depressive symptoms and severity of the depressive episode also correlate with recurrence. Suicidality and a need for psychiatric admission weigh heavily in the decision surrounding maintenance because recurrence carries even greater risks of suicide for the patient. Comorbid medical or psychiatric diagnoses not only complicate treatment but also increase the risk of recurrence. However, the most important factor may be patient preference. Despite a high risk of recurrence, some patients insist on trying a period of time without medications. Fully understanding patients' reasons may uncover their significant side effects or false perceptions about mental illness that can be addressed. If the patient still decides to discontinue treatment, then it is important for the clinician and the patient to monitor for early signs of recurrence and have a plan in place.

When maintenance therapy is used, it is typically continued indefinitely. The same dose used to achieve remission is maintained and not decreased for maintenance treatment. There is growing evidence to suggest that psychotherapy combined with medications decreases the risk for recurrence. Some patients have done well with psychotherapy alone after gradual cessation of medications during the maintenance phase. We currently recommend neither decreasing nor stopping medications in maintenance-phase treatment but strongly suggest considering the addition of psychotherapy to the patient's treatment regimen. However, for those patients who strongly prefer to try stopping antidepressant medication, continuing psychotherapy may reduce the risk of relapse.

■ Initial Treatment Strategies

Medications are most frequently the initial intervention used by clinicians today for the treatment of depression. However, strong evidence also supports the use of psychotherapy as initial monotherapy, despite its frequent relegation to second-line treatment.

Psychotherapy

Psychotherapy is often overlooked as a treatment option for patients with major depression or dysthymia. There is strong evidence of its efficacy as monotherapy in both mild to moderate depression and dysthymia and as an adjunctive therapy in severe and chronic forms of depression. Adjunctive psychotherapy is usually helpful and recommended when the patient is willing. It is an especially important consideration if initial treatment fails to achieve a full remission (see Chapter 5). Today most clinicians recommend that initial treatment for dysthymia include an antidepressant and psychotherapy, though patients' preferences influence the actual treatment choices. Like recurrent major depression, dysthymia's treatment is almost always long-term.

The subject of psychotherapy is enormous and has a long history dating back to before Sigmund Freud. In an effort to condense and simplify this topic, we have focused our discussion in this section on information that will help the general clinician recognize appropriate situations for recommending psychotherapy as an *initial* treatment for depression. Other sections in the book will discuss psychotherapy as it pertains to that section's focus—exposure therapy for phobias, a combination of psychotherapy and medications in treatment-resistant depression, and so on.

■ Background

Empirical study of psychotherapies has been challenging because the techniques of many psychotherapies are hard to standardize, the conditions that the psychotherapies treat are often heterogeneous, and the effects or outcomes of the psychotherapies can be difficult to quantify and measure. The difficulties encountered when studying psychotherapies do not negate the benefits that many people have experienced with many types of psychotherapy; rather, these difficulties make it harder to understand precisely *why* and *how* people benefit from these treatments. Over the last 2 decades, one particular form of psychotherapy, cognitive behavioral therapy (CBT), has been front and center in psychotherapy research for several reasons: (1) the focus is on more easily measured behaviors and thoughts as opposed to insight about feelings; (2) the techniques of CBT are very specific and easily standardized into a manual; and (3) it was initially developed for patients with a definable disorder (e.g., depression). For these reasons, we will focus most of our attention about psychotherapy on CBT for the initial treatment of depression.

CBT, as conceived by Aaron Beck, views personality and psychopathology as sets of assumptions or cognitive schemas that are created in response to an individual's significant experiences and social learning. These schemas are then used by the individual to evaluate events (i.e., perceptions) and organize responses (i.e., behaviors) that fit within the cognitive schemas. In health, an individual's cognitive schemas are adaptive and synergistic with overall functioning and health. In some psychiatric disorders (Beck first focused on depression), the "disordered" (e.g., depressed) cognitive schema maintains cognitions of sadness, loss, and hopelessness. Beck hypothesized that altering or modifying the cognitive schemas and behaviors associated with depression would relieve the symptoms caused by depression. CBT was first developed as a short-term (i.e., 12 sessions) treatment for depression that focused on identifying the "depressed" cognitive schemas and behaviors, then modifying them with the help of a psychotherapist. With the development of new, "not depressed" cognitive schemas and behaviors the symptoms of depression abated. Unlike psychodynamic psychotherapies, developing insight regarding *why* these thoughts and behaviors exist is *not* necessary for recovery.

CBT is conceptualized by many as a series of highly specific patient-centered learning experiences that are guided and facilitated by a psychotherapist trained in CBT. The learning experiences teach the patient different operations, including the following:

- Identify and monitor negative, automatic thoughts.
- Recognize how thoughts, feelings, and behaviors interact and affect each other. This interaction is the basis of a cognitive schema.

■ Confront the distorted cognition (i.e., cognitive schema) with reality-based evidence from current experience.

■ Insert reality-based observations into the cognitive schema and then test them out.

This is a vast oversimplification, but most patients easily grasp these basic constructs. Their understanding of and comfort with the process of psychotherapy is the key to acceptance and adherence. The literature supports the use of CBT in the acute and maintenance phases of treatment for depression. Its role in combined treatments (e.g., CBT plus medication) is discussed in the next chapter, which focuses on treatment approaches for depression when the initial treatment is inadequate.

The American Psychiatric Association's *Practice Guideline for the Treatment of Patients with Major Depressive Disorder* recommends that CBT be a monotherapy treatment in the acute-phase treatment for only mild to moderate depression (2). Others have argued that CBT is as effective as medications in patients with severe depression, but the data for this assertion is less decisive.

Though there is some evidence that supports CBT as a monotherapy in the acute phase of treatment for more serious depression, there is greater evidence to support its use in combination with medication when dealing with more complex depression (i.e., chronic depression, residual symptoms, recurrent episodes, comorbid conditions) in acute and especially maintenance phases of treatment (see Chapter 5).

■ Comanagement with a Therapist

Shared treatment arrangements—in which a general clinician provides ongoing general care that could include pharmacotherapy and a psychotherapist provides psychotherapy—have become increasingly more common. Clear communication between the general clinician, patient, and psychotherapist about expectations and roles provides the best possible chance for a successful treatment outcome. This is true not only with psychotherapists but also with other shared treatment relationships involving other specialists (e.g., cardiologists, neurologists, surgeons).

■ Pharmacotherapy

The pharmaceutical industry has focused much of our attention on the differences between antidepressants. However, *all* of the current antidepressant agents are equally efficacious in treating depression when compared to a placebo. Though the differences between antidepressants are important, the practices of adequate dosing and length of treatment with an antidepressant are of much greater importance. When antidepressants are compared at full dosages after 12 weeks, there is essentially no difference in response and remission rates. In general, response rates to an initial antidepressant vary between 40% and 60%. This variation is most likely due to population differences, severity of depression, and study design, not the agents. Conversely, 40% to 60% of patients treated for depression will not respond to the first agent. Currently, the pharmacotherapy approach to depression is similar to the drug treatment of hypertension; that is, *serial monotherapies are attempted first, and augmenting agents or additional drugs are added when only partial responses occur.* The decision of which agent to choose is based on matching the agent's likely effects and side effects (e.g., sedation, stimulation, GI upset) with the patient's target symptoms (e.g., insomnia, fatigue) and particular patient concerns (e.g., weight gain, sexual side effects). Though initially the clinician is striving to find a match for the patient and their unique symptoms, the greater emphasis should remain on utilizing a full dosage, an adequate period of time, and, of course, patient compliance.

■ Discontinuation Syndrome

Antidepressants should not be suddenly discontinued. Abrupt cessation or interruption after continual use for 4 or more weeks with any antidepressant can result in a *discontinuation syndrome.* All of the tricyclic antidepressants (TCAs) have been associated with this syndrome. Those selective serotonin reuptake inhibitors (SSRIs) and serotonin-norepinephrine reuptake inhibitors (SNRIs) that have shorter half-lives and few or no active metabolites (i.e., paroxetine and venlafaxine) are usually associated with discontinuation syndromes; fluoxetine has the least association with discontinuation syndromes because of its long half-life.

Symptoms can include acute anxiety, depressed mood, sleep disturbances, paresthesias, dizziness, nausea, vomiting, diarrhea headaches, tremor, ataxia, and sweating. Discontinuation syndrome is *not* "serotonin syndrome," which is due to excessive drug effects and is potentially life-threatening. Discontinuation syndromes are unpleasant but not life-threatening. Management is either to reinstitute the antidepressant or a similar agent or to use supportive measures until the symptoms abate in several days.

Limitations of Neurotransmitter Theories
No single reproducible biological abnormality in any neurotransmitter or its receptors has been shown to cause major depression or any other psychiatric disorder. Psychiatry has generally shifted away from the pursuit of a single biological reason to explain depression (i.e., biological reductionism); instead, psychiatry emphasizes and defines all of the variables that

contribute to the risk of a psychiatric disorder. Currently, psychiatric disorders are believed to result from the complex interaction between inherited genetic factors, acquired gene activation or inactivation, life experiences, one's thoughts and behaviors, and social circumstances. Ultimately, these all interact and result in some change in the central nervous system's (CNS) neurotransmitter systems. Medications do change the levels of neurotransmitters in the CNS, but we urge caution in assuming that a medication's effect on these neurotransmitters accounts for treatment success or failure.

Major Antidepressant Classes

As noted previously, the clinician's task is to match an antidepressant's predicted effects and side effects with the patient's target symptoms and preferences. The classes of antidepressants and their profiles are reviewed in Box 4-2. For each antidepressant class, we will describe the presumed mode of action, starting doses, maximum doses, major side effects, and unique properties that would suggest its benefit in certain clinical situations (e.g., bupropion to avoid weight gain). The world of antidepressants continues to evolve, and new agents are always in the pipeline. As new agents come out and pharmaceutical representatives sing their praises, remember that the particular antidepressant chosen is less important than taking it to its full dosage for an adequate period of time.

> **Box 4-2 Major Antidepressant Classes**
>
> - Tricyclic antidepressants (TCAs)
> - Selective serotonin reuptake inhibitors (SSRIs)
> - Serotonin-norepinephrine reuptake inhibitors (SNRIs)
> - Other agents (e.g., bupropion, mirtazapine, trazodone, nefazodone)
> - Monoamine oxidase inhibitors (MAOIs)

Tricyclic Antidepressants

Like forgotten older antibiotics, TCAs (see Box 4-3) are not typically considered as first-line therapy, yet they have a long record of experience and evidence of efficacy. Prior to the 1990s, these agents were the mainstay of the treatment of depression for over 30 years. Imipramine was first tested

> **Box 4-3 Tricyclic Antidepressants**
>
> Amitriptyline (Elavil)
> Clomipramine (Anafranil)
> Desipramine (Norpramin)
> Imipramine (Tofranil)
> Nortriptyline (Pamelor, Aventil)

in 1958 as an antipsychotic and ultimately as an antidepressant. The TCAs as a class have similar effects and side effects. They block the reuptake of norepinephrine, serotonin, and to a lesser degree, dopamine. Their side effects are primarily derived from the blockade of muscarinic cholinergic receptors, H1 histamine receptors, and alpha-1-adrenergic receptors.

The majority of TCAs primarily block the reuptake of norepinephrine. Clomipramine (Anafranil) stands out as an exception because it has a high

Table 4-1 Characteristics and Dosage of Tricyclic Antidepressants

Tricyclic Antidepressants	Dry Mouth, Constipation	Sedation	Weight Gain	Orthostatic Hypotension	Sexual Dysfunction	Drug-Drug Interactions	Starting Dose (mg)	Usual Daily Dose (mg)
Amitriptyline	+++	++++	+++	+++	+++	All TCAs are metabolized in the liver; all are substrates, and none are potent inhibitors or inducers	25	25-300
Clomipramine	++	++	++	++			50	75-300
Desipramine	++	+	++	++			50	75-200
Imipramine	+++	+++	++++	+++			50	50-300
Nortriptyline	++	++	+	++			25	50-150

+ = magnitude of side effect

affinity for serotonin receptors. Of note is the fact that clomipramine's active metabolite, *N*-desmethylclomipramine, is a potent norepinephrine reuptake inhibitor. Clomipramine is used primarily to treat obsessive-compulsive disorder (OCD) and represents the link between TCAs and the more recently developed SSRIs.

Despite the potential for lethal overdose (see discussion under TCA Overdose), TCAs remain a good choice for the treatment of depression. Patients who have insomnia, pain, or poor appetite may be good candidates for a TCA. The authors most frequently use nortriptyline because it is the least anticholinergic and is the only antidepressant with a defined therapeutic window in serum levels. Imipramine levels have also been correlated with response, but a therapeutic window has not been established. For nortriptyline, the level vs response curve is an inverted "U." Nortriptyline levels provide especially valuable information in patients for whom absorption, metabolism, or compliance is a concern. It is important to note that *decreasing* the dose when the nortriptyline level is above 150 ng/mL may *increase* the response.

The typical starting dose of nortriptyline is 10 to 25 mg taken at night, and it is slowly titrated up. Levels are usually collected when a steady state is achieved or when there are side effects. One caveat is that nortriptyline levels are confounded in medical conditions where alpha-1 acid glycoprotein (an acute phase reactant), the primary plasma protein to which TCAs bind, is increased or decreased.

Amitriptyline and imipramine are more sedating and have more anticholinergic effects than the other TCAs (e.g., nortriptyline, desipramine). Amitriptyline is the parent compound of nortriptyline, and imipramine is the parent compound of desipramine. Amitriptyline and imipramine are currently not frequently used as monotherapy because they are not well tolerated at effective doses. Amitriptyline is frequently used to treat chronic neuropathic pain with or without depression. The burden of side effects and drug-drug interactions limit much higher doses.

TCA Overdose

The major drawback to TCAs is their risk for toxicity and potential lethality in overdose. TCAs block sodium channels in the heart and brain, which can cause cardiac arrhythmias and seizures. TCA overdose is a medical emergency and requires immediate intervention. Cardiac complications of TCA overdose (i.e., heart block, ventricular tachycardia and fibrillation, asystole and cardiogenic shock) are fortunately relatively infrequent. In 2 reviews of consecutive admissions to the ICU for TCA overdose, the rates of serious arrhythmias ranged from 3 of 225 (1.3%) to 4 of 153 patients (2.6%), whereas significant hypotension ranged from 14% to 51%. In another case series, coma was an ominous sign, present in 53 of 316 overdoses (17%) but present in 53% of overdoses that were ultimately fatal. Management is most frequently supportive and should include cardiac monitoring. Gastric lavage should be limited to cases in which ingestion occurred less than 1 hour prior to lavage (3). Activated charcoal is routinely given, but it is hard to reduce the absorption of TCAs from the gut. When a cardiac arrhythmia or hypotension is present, alkalinization with sodium bicarbonate *or* hyperventilation is helpful. Combining both may cause excessive alkalinization. In general, antiarrhythmic drugs should be avoided because interventions targeted at correcting hypotension, acidosis, and hypoxia are more effective in reducing TCAs' effects on the myocardium, and some antiarrhythmic drugs can make the arrhythmia worse (e.g., quinidine, procainamide, bretylium, amiodarone). Lidocaine and beta-blockers have been cautiously used with some success.

Adverse Effects

All TCAs possess type IC antiarrhythmic activity. The Cardiac Arrhythmia Suppression Trial (CAST) found that type IC antiarrhythmic drugs given following myocardial infarction may increase the risk of sudden death (4). TCAs may pose similar risks. If TCAs are used in patients who have a history of heart disease, particularly conduction abnormalities, or are at a higher risk for cardiac arrhythmias (e.g., the elderly), a pretreatment electrocardiogram (EKG) should be obtained and followed periodically.

Selective Serotonin Reuptake Inhibitors

Currently, the most common first-line pharmacotherapy treatment for depression is with an SSRI (see Box 4-4). As compared to TCAs, SSRIs are generally less sedating, less likely to cause weight gain, and are nonlethal in overdose. Most SSRIs do not have noticeable effects on depression for upward of 3 to 6 weeks after initiating therapy and, not uncommonly, require 6 to 7 weeks to see a response. The SSRI's safety in overdose is a key advantage in the treatment of depression and other psychiatric disorders with increased risk for suicide.

> **Box 4-4 Selective Serotonin Reuptake Inhibitors**
>
> Citalopram (Celexa)
> Escitalopram (Lexapro)
> Fluoxetine (Prozac)
> Fluvoxamine (Luvox)
> Paroxetine (Paxil, Paxil CR)
> Sertraline (Zoloft)

Both TCAs and SSRIs are equally likely to cause sexual dysfunction. That said, SSRIs carry their own side-effect burdens, and the choice of SSRI, like TCA, is based on matching effect and side-effect profiles with the unique characteristics of the patient (e.g., target symptoms, comorbidities). All SSRIs are equally effective in the treatment of depression. All selectively block serotonin reuptake thereby increasing the amount of serotonin available in the synapse. All are hepatically metabolized through the cytochrome P450 systems. In addition to being substrates, some SSRIs significantly inhibit specific cytochrome systems causing drug-drug interactions. As a group, SSRI side effects include sexual dysfunction, GI upset, headache, sleep disturbance, and fatigue. There are some differences between the agents when looked at across large cohorts of patients; those differences are noted in Table 4-2. The SSRIs' role as "first-line" pharmacotherapy is currently challenged by other new antidepressants (e.g., venlafaxine, duloxetine, bupropion, and mirtazapine), some of which are discussed in the following table.

Starting at low doses and gradually increasing the dosage minimizes the side effects frequently associated with the initiation of an SSRI (e.g., agitation, GI upset). Typically, initial side effects abate during the first 2 weeks. Sexual side effects are associated with all of these agents and seem to be dose related. This is discussed in greater detail in the following section.

Adverse Effects

SSRIs can induce initial insomnia despite their ability to normalize middle insomnia that is frequently seen with major depression. This can be managed by either switching to a morning dosing schedule or adding a sedative hypnotic at night. Trazodone works particularly well in this case, but other agents, such as temazepam and zolpidem, are useful, too. Though SSRIs are not associated with severe cardiac side effects like the TCAs, SSRIs can cause bradycardia in rare cases.

Serotonin syndrome, which results from very high levels of serotonin, is fortunately uncommon but potentially life-threatening when it occurs. It is characterized by extreme gastrointestinal distress (e.g., nausea and vomiting), altered mental status (e.g., irritability, confusion, delirium), hyperreflexia, myoclonus, ataxia, and autonomic instability (e.g., hyperthermia, hypertension, tachycardia, diaphoresis). Serotonin syndrome typically occurs when 2 or more serotonergic agents are given either concurrently or before adequate washout (e.g., when other antidepressants overlap with MAOIs). There can be some overlap between the hypertensive crises associated with MAOIs and serotonin syndrome. Hypertensive crisis is associated

Table 4-2 Characteristics and Dosages of SSRIs

SSRI	Sedation	Weight Gain	Sexual Dysfunction	Starting Dose (mg)	Usual Daily Dose (mg)
Citalopram	+/-	+	++	20	20-60
Escitalopram	-	+	++	10	10-40
Fluvoxamine*	+	+	++	25	100-200
Fluoxetine	--	+/-	++	10-20	20-60
Paroxetine	++	++	+++	20	20-60
Sertraline	+/-	+	++	25-50	50-200

*Fluvoxamine is used twice daily; all other SSRIs have once-daily dosing.
+ = magnitude of side effect; - = no problem

with MAOIs and norepinephrine elevations, whereas serotonin syndrome involves serotonin. Agents that increase availability of both norepinephrine and serotonin (i.e., TCAs and SNRIs) can produce a mixed picture of hypertensive crisis and serotonin syndrome. Typically, 2 weeks are needed to wash out most antidepressants before initiating an MAOI. Fluoxetine requires up to 6 weeks because of its long half-life and active metabolites. There are other agents that are not antidepressants that still have significant serotonergic activity and can cause serotonin syndrome when mixed with most antidepressants; these agents include tramadol (Ultram), triptans, and cocaine. Serotonin syndrome is often self-limited and resolves with supportive care and cessation of the offending agents, but some symptom reduction may be achieved by administering cyproheptadine (Periactin).

Serotonin-Norepinephrine Reuptake Inhibitors

Duloxetine (Cymbalta) and Venlafaxine (Effexor)

Selective serotonin-norepinephrine reuptake inhibitors (SNRIs) include duloxetine (Cymbalta) and venlafaxine (Effexor) (see Table 4-3). Safety, tolerability, and side-effect profiles are similar to that of the SSRIs, with the exception of some SNRIs that have been associated with a sustained rise in blood pressure at higher doses. In clinical trials, venlafaxine increased diastolic blood pressure by >15 mm Hg in 5.5% of patients at dosages above 200 mg per day. Duloxetine increased diastolic blood pressure by an average of 1 mm Hg in 5% of patients with dosages between 60 and 120 mg, but a minority of patients have more significant increases. Nausea is a more frequent side effect with SNRIs (venlafaxine [37%] and duloxetine [35% to 40%]) than SSRIs in general (20% to 26%). SNRIs can be used as first-line agents, particularly in patients with significant fatigue or pain syndromes associated with the episode of depression. The SNRIs also have an important role as second-line agents in patients who have not responded to SSRIs.

Other Antidepressants

Bupropion (Wellbutrin) is a norepinephrine and dopamine reuptake inhibitor. It can cause seizures at high dosages and, according to the Food and Drug Administration (FDA), is contraindicated in patients with a history of bulimia or anorexia nervosa (AN). Bupropion's risk for seizures should not be overestimated. It was initially prescribed at doses of 600 to 800 mg per day, and one study in women with bulimia found a 4% risk of seizures. More recent information shows the risk of seizures to gradually increase from 0.1% (100-300 mg/day) to 0.4% (300-450 mg/day) and ultimately 2.3% (>600 mg/day); the baseline risk for new-onset seizures is 0.06%. Most patients respond to 300 mg per day, and doses above 450 mg are rarely used. Bupropion is unique among antidepressants because it neither causes sexual dysfunction nor weight gain, and it also aids smoking cessation. Side effects include dizziness, weight loss, dry mouth, and agitation. Some patients

Table 4-3 Characteristics and Dosage of SNRIs and Other Antidepressant Agents

	Sedation	Weight Gain	Cardiac	Sexual Dysfunction	Starting Dose (mg)	Usual Daily Dose (mg)
SNRIs						
Venlafaxine XR	-	+	+ Elevated heart rate and blood pressure	++	37.5	150-300
Duloxetine	-	+	+/-	++	30	60-120
Other Agents						
Bupropion	-	-	+ Elevated blood pressure	-	100	300-400
Mirtazapine	++	+++	-	-	15	45-60
Trazodone	+++	++	+ Decreased blood pressure	Rare priapism	25-50	100-300
Nefazodone	+	-	-	-	50	300-500

+ = magnitude of side effect; - = no problem

experience increased heart rate and elevated blood pressure, but this is uncommon. However, when bupropion is used in conjunction with a nicotine patch, the incidence of elevated blood pressure has been about 6%.

Mirtazapine (Remeron) is another useful antidepressant. Though its mechanism of action is not fully delineated, it increases serotonin and norepinephrine in the CNS and is also an alpha-2 antagonist. Its most common side effects, weight gain and sedation, are due mostly to its antihistaminic effect. Both of these side effects may decrease with acclimation to higher doses. A soluble tablet form is available, which is useful in patients who cannot swallow pills. Though mirtazapine is not typically a first-line treatment for depression, it is a particularly good choice in a patient who has significant anorexia or insomnia. It also seems useful in patients who have mixed depression with anxiety symptoms. Typically, 15 mg is initiated at bedtime and titrated up by 15 mg increments.

Trazodone's (Desyrel) mechanisms of action are not well delineated, but it is presumed to block the serotonin postsynaptic receptor, and its active metabolite works like a weak SSRI. For most patients, trazodone is effective as an antidepressant at doses of 300 mg and above. Trazodone is usually not considered a first-line treatment for depression because adequate dosage tends to be too sedating, explaining its frequent use as a sleep aid (see Chapter 3). Trazodone's starting dosage range is 25 to 50 mg. It can be titrated up slowly by 25-50 mg every 3 to 5 days until an adequate response is achieved. Part of the reason for the initially slow titration of trazodone is that it can cause postural hypotension, especially if started at higher doses. Trazodone can rarely cause priapism, occurring once in 6000 men and less often in women (i.e., clitoral priapism). Some clinicians unnecessarily avoid its use because of an overestimation of the risk. It is prudent to warn male patients about this rare adverse effect and what to do if it occurs.

Nefazodone is much less sedating than trazodone, and for this reason it is better tolerated at antidepressant dosages. It also does not cause priapism and has less postural hypotension (3%). Bristol-Myers Squibb discontinued sales of nefazodone (Serzone) effective June 2004 because of safety concerns regarding life-threatening hepatic failure. The risk is calculated to be about 30 in 100,000. It is metabolized through CYP450 3A4, so extra caution is warranted if co-administered drugs are also metabolized through this system. Nefazodone is still available in its generic form.

Monoamine Oxidase Inhibitors

MAOIs (i.e., tranylcypramine, phenelzine), developed in the 1950s, were the first effective therapy for depression. However, because of their interactions with certain drugs and foods resulting in hypertensive crisis (see Box 4-5), they were quickly eclipsed by TCAs. In current times, only psychiatrists prescribe MAOIs for patients with refractory, treatment-resistant depression. Though general clinicians rarely encounter patients on MAOI antidepressants, it is important to emphasize that there are 2 serious adverse reactions associated with MAOIs: hypertensive crises and serotonin syndrome (discussed earlier in this chapter). Hypertensive crises occur when catecholamines reach dangerous levels because an MAOI blocks their metabolism by the inhibiting monoamine oxidase enzyme. This state can occur by ingesting a sympathomimetic medication, taking a medication that

> **Box 4-5 Examples of Dangerous Interactions with MAOIs**
>
> - Tyramine-rich foods (e.g., aged foods, wine, cheese; see the Appendix for a detailed list of foods)
> - Serotonergic agents
> - Meperidine (Demerol)
> - Nonselective sympathomimetics (e.g., pseudoephedrine)
> - Stimulants
> - Other antidepressants

inhibits reuptake of norepinephrine (e.g., TCAs, SNRIs), or eating catecholamine-rich (tyramine) foods while taking an MAOI. This is a medical emergency because severe hypertension leading to seizures, stroke, and even death can occur. The management includes stopping the offending agent or agents, reducing blood pressure (but not with betablockers, which would leave alpha-adrenergic effects unopposed), and initiating supportive care.

Seligeline is an MAOI initially approved for Parkinson disease and was recently released in the United States as a transdermal patch. It has been shown to be safe and effective in treating major depression. It is unique as an antidepressant because it is available as a transdermal patch, providing the only practical option for treating depression in typically hospitalized patients who must take nothing by mouth for a long period. At low doses, seligeline is a relatively selective MAOI because it inhibits MAO-B but not MAO-A. Hence, when used at the lowest dose (6 mg) the manufacturer states that no dietary restrictions are required as with other MAOIs. At higher doses of 9 and 12 mg, selectivity may be lost, and dietary and medication restrictions are required.

Stimulants

The stimulants D-amphetamine (Dexedrine) and methylphenidate (Ritalin) can be used as a monotherapy, as an initial treatment until an antidepressant starts to have its effects, and in combination with an antidepressant in the long term. They are particularly useful as an initial treatment in debilitated and medically ill patients, in whom one cannot wait the 6 to 8 weeks for a response that traditional antidepressants require. Stimulants are also used in patients with residual depressive symptoms. See Chapter 5 for a complete discussion of stimulants, including a detailed discussion of their use as initial treatment in debilitated and medically ill patients.

Matching Target Symptoms with Side-Effect Profiles of Antidepressants

Insomnia and Hypersomnolence

Depression may cause insomnia or hypersomnolence, as can some antidepressants. Antidepressants have diverse, complex effects on sleep laboratory measures, but the clinical significance of these measures is not entirely clear. Randomized controlled trials have shown mixed results. For example, one comparing nefazodone vs fluoxetine showed that both are equally effective as antidepressants, but nefazodone is less disruptive of sleep (5). Another study comparing imipramine versus fluoxetine also found that both were equally effective as antidepressants, but both equally improved baseline insomnia. Baseline insomnia did not predict any difference in response to either antidepressant (6). When all SSRIs are considered, insomnia occurs as a side-effect in about 10% to 20% of patients, and while drowsiness is not common (<5%), for some individual patients it may be profound. Trazodone and nefazodone cause no more insomnia than a placebo, but they cause drowsiness in 25% of patients.

For chronic insomnia, sleep hygiene is also important (e.g., keeping a regular bedtime, avoiding nonsleeping activity in bed, avoiding naps, eliminating caffeine). Persistent insomnia should also raise suspicion of bipolar illness, substance abuse, or sleep apnea. For information about treating depression with insomnia, see Box 4-6.

Some patients' daytime hypersomnolence appears to be a consequence of nighttime insomnia. For them, the strategies in Box 4-6 are appropriate. For those with hypersomnolence without insomnia, clinical experience supports the strategies in Box 4-7. If hypersomnolence persists after resolution of other depressive symptoms, the patient should be evaluated for other causes, such as narcolepsy or sleep apnea.

Box 4-6 Strategies for Depression with Insomnia

- Avoid using stimulating antidepressants (e.g. bupropion).
- Use or add a sedating antidepressant (e.g., trazodone, mirtazapine).
- Add a hypnotic (e.g., zolpidem).

Box 4-7 Strategies for Depression with Hypersomnolence

- Use a stimulating antidepressant (e.g., bupropion) taken in the morning.
- Add a stimulant to the antidepressant.

■ Sexual Dysfunction

In a recent study, 60% to 70% of patients treated with SSRIs experienced associated sexual dysfunction. Sexual dysfunction can range from decreased libido, to decreased arousal, to difficulty achieving orgasm (see Figure 4-3). Serotonin is involved in all 3 phases of sexual functioning. Identifying the primary phase disrupted will help determine appropriate interventions.

There are few randomized, placebo-controlled trials to guide the treatment of SSRI-associated sexual dysfunction. Placebo response rates in clinical trials have been high (up to 60%). Also, there is significant sexual dysfunction associated with depression itself that often reverses with antidepressant treatment. Given this complexity, the first step is a careful assessment with a history that focuses on pretreatment of sexual functioning, the phase that is primarily disturbed, and other causes of sexual dysfunction. Educating the patient about the relevance of this information is critical to the formulation of a treatment plan. This information explains that prolonged time for arousal may be needed or that sexual functioning may improve after time with acclimation to the medication. A 1-day drug holiday or a weekend reduction of dosage is also frequently helpful.

In the event that the management detailed in Box 4-8 fails and the sexual side effect persists, then switching agents or pharmacologic intervention may be necessary. Bupropion and nefazodone have sexual dysfunction rates close to a placebo in drug trials. Mirtazapine has more associated sexual dysfunction than a placebo but less than SSRIs. Randomized trial data support the use of sildenafil in men with

> **Box 4-8 Management of Sexual Dysfunction in Patients Using SSRIs**
>
> 1. Take a careful history. Identify the primary phase disturbed and rule out other causes.
> 2. Educate the patient about the response to be expected.
> 3. Wait for adaptation.
> 4. Alter the dosing schedule by reducing the dose or taking a drug holiday.
> 5. Switch antidepressants.
> 6. Try pharmacologic treatments, such as bupropion or sildenafil.

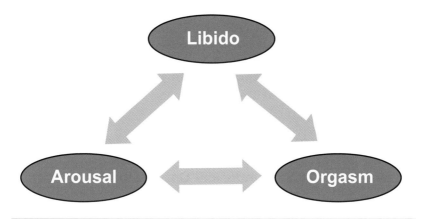

Figure 4-3

SSRI-associated sexual dysfunction. A few case reports (but no randomized clinical trial data) support the use of sildenafil in women with SSRI-induced sexual dysfunction. Substitution of an SSRI with bupropion is helpful for some patients with problems of reduced libido or delayed arousal, but there is conflicting evidence about whether bupropion can reverse SSRI-induced sexual dysfunction when co-administered (1 positive open trial, 1 negative RCT). Other agents (e.g., yohimbine, methylphenidate, amantadine) have been reported as effective, but the benefits have not materialized in clinical trials.

Weight Gain

Weight gain is seen with SSRIs but is much more common with TCAs and mirtazapine. The increase is most often limited to the first 3 months of treatment and usually requires little or no intervention. It is difficult to sort out what is an effect vs a side effect of medications during the acute phase because weight and appetite changes are common symptoms of depression. However, changing the agent is reasonable when weight gain continues after acute-phase treatment despite remission or weight gain is significant (5%-10% above the patient's ideal body weight) and when conservative measures of increased exercise and decreased caloric intake have failed. Bupropion or nefazodone are less likely to affect weight than the SSRIs. Of the SSRIs, fluoxetine is associated with weight loss in some patients.

Anorexia Nervosa

For anorexia nervosa (AN), clinical experience and reported side effects in clinical trials would favor appetite-stimulating antidepressants (e.g., mirtazapine, TCAs) over antidepressants that sometimes cause AN and weight loss (e.g., fluoxetine, bupropion). The index of suspicion is raised for AN in the young female patient with major depression and AN. The approach to AN with major depression is reviewed in Chapter 16.

Electroconvulsive Therapy

Electroconvulsive therapy (ECT) is another important consideration in the treatment of severe depression where rapid reduction of symptoms (e.g., severe malnutrition, active suicidal intent, psychosis, catatonia, pregnancy) is imperative. ECT is discussed in detail in Chapter 5, where its use in refractory depression is outlined.

■ Treatments for Adjunctive Therapy in Major Depression and the Management of Mood Symptoms in Subsyndromal Depression

The symptomatic management of subsyndromal depressive disorders covers a broad range of interventions, including pharmacologic, psychotherapeutic, behavioral, social, and lifestyle interventions (see Table 4-4). The patient's preference is the primary consideration in choosing the intervention. Often a prescribed intervention is not warranted because the "psychotherapy" performed during the initial visit may be the only intervention required. Most nonpsychiatric clinicians do not characterize their interactions with patients as psychotherapy. However, identifying stressors, labeling symptoms as syndromes (i.e., disorders), identifying adaptive and maladaptive coping strategies, problem solving, and reflective listening are all tools of effective psychotherapy and are components of effective interviewing. When symptoms persist or the psychosocial stressor is complex (e.g., job loss, severe medical illness, disaster survival), psychotherapy performed by a skilled therapist is an important intervention. Other nonpharmacologic interventions include exercise, cessation of psychoactive substances, sleep hygiene, nutrition, religious involvement, and education.

Pharmacologic Treatment of Subsyndromal Depression

Symptomatic pharmacologic interventions include trazodone, sedative-hypnotics, benzodiazepines, and analgesics. Sleep, pain, and anxiety are the most commonly targeted symptoms. These agents are all familiar to general clinicians, except perhaps trazodone. Though technically an antidepressant, at lower doses it is an effective sleeping aid (although the database is sparse for trazodone's sedative-hypnotic use). It is available in a generic form, can be used long term, and is not addictive or abused; it is widely used for patients who need a medication for more than initial insomnia. Trazodone's starting dosage range is 25-50 mg. It can be titrated up slowly at a rate of 25-50 mg every 3 to 5 days until adequate response. Part of the reason for the initially slow titration of trazodone is that it can cause hypotension if started at higher doses. This side effect seldom occurs when started at low dose and titrated up as noted. For many, the starting dose is often adequate, and no increase is required. Morning sedation is common at doses more than 100-150mg. Adjusting dosage and taking it earlier in the evening are common alterations to trazodone therapy to reduce the morning "hangover." Priapism is a very rare complication, occurring

Table 4-4 Symptomatic Management of Subsyndromal Depression	
Nonpharmacologic	*Pharmacologic*
Psychotherapy	Hypnotics (e.g., zolpidem)
Exercise	Benzodiazepines (e.g., clonazepam)
Nutrition	Analgesics (e.g., acetaminophen, NSAIDs)
Religious involvement	Phosphodiesterase inhibitors (e.g., sildenafil, vardenafil)
Reduction of psychoactive agents	
St. John's wort	
Patient education	

once in 6000 men and less often in women (i.e., clitoral priapism). Some clinicians unnecessarily avoid its use because of an overestimation of the risk. It is prudent to warn male patients about this rare adverse effect and what to do if it occurs.

Benzodiazepines are typically associated with anxiety disorders; however, anxiety symptoms are frequently a component of depressive disorders, including subsyndromal depression. Short-term benzodiazepine use is particularly effective when patients "can't stop thinking about" a recent event (e.g., death, illness in a loved one) or are having trouble "turning off" their minds to go to sleep. Though sedative hypnotics (discussed in the next paragraph) work well for initial insomnia, they have little daytime effect. When benzodiazepines are prescribed, longer-acting benzodiazepines (e.g., clonazepam) are preferred over short-acting and rapid-acting benzodiazepines (e.g., alprazolam), because longer-acting agents used at night may have mild antianxiety effects during the day, are easier to taper off, and are less likely to be misused or abused than benzodiazepines. Typical starting doses for clonazepam are 0.25 mg to 0.5 mg at bedtime or twice daily.

Sedative-hypnotic medications are useful when sleep hygiene interventions (see Sleep Hygiene later in this chapter) have failed. Transient initial insomnia is common in periods of increased stress that may be accompanied by depressive symptoms. Typically, an agent suitable for initial insomnia (e.g., zolpidem) is prescribed for short-term use. Chronic use of sedative-hypnotic drugs should be avoided because they are CNS depressants and may lead to dependency and withdrawal, making them particularly risky in patients with current or prior substance abuse. Even though the newer sedative agents are technically "nonnarcotic" and should carry a lower abuse potential, caution is still warranted. If chronic therapy for insomnia is needed, then trazodone is often used.

Analgesics are important to consider when dealing with depressive syndromes. Pain can make depressive symptoms worse, and the converse is also true. In addition, both depression and pain aggravate—and are aggravated by—insomnia. Given the scope and complexity of this topic, the discussion of pain, depression, and its treatment are beyond the goals of this section (7). For the discussion here, the clinician is reminded to ask about pain and fully evaluate it. Nonnarcotic analgesics (e.g., nonsteroidal anti-inflammatory drugs [NSAIDs] and acetaminophen) are relatively safe and simple interventions. Physical therapy, occupational therapy, and exercise programs (discussed later in this chapter) can all have a significant impact on pain reduction and subsequent depressive symptoms.

Drugs for Erectile Dysfunction

Depression and erectile dysfunction (ED) commonly occur together in men, but the causal relationship is often unclear. Erectile dysfunction is twice as likely in men suffering from depression than those who are not. Which came first, ED or depressive symptoms, is less clear. ED can be a symptom of major depression that resolves with treatment of the depression. Sexual side effects are common with most antidepressants in both men and women (see Chapter 6). The association is less defined in men with ED and subsyndromal depression. The effects of sildenafil were evaluated among men with ED and mild-to-moderate depressive symptoms in a randomized, double-blind, placebo-controlled, flexible-dose (25-100 mg) trial over 12 weeks. Patients had only mild depression; those meeting criteria for major depression were excluded. ED, orgasmic function, sexual desire, and over-all satisfaction with intercourse improved significantly more in the sildenafil group (P < 0.001 for all comparisons). The other phosphodiesterase inhibitors, tadalafil (Cialis) and vardenafil (Levitra), have not been studied in this manner to date.

Nonpharmacological Interventions

Patients with subsyndromal depressive symptoms frequently prefer non-pharmacological interventions. These interventions may be also combined with antidepressants (when major depression is present) and psychother-apy. Some adjunctive interventions have been demonstrated as beneficial, while others remain unproven but potentially helpful.

Exercise

Depression rates are lower in physically active patients, and generally depressed patients are more physically inactive as a result of the depres-sion itself. Exercise in almost any form (e.g., aerobic and less intense forms) is an effective adjunct in the treatment of depression, improving energy, mood, appetite, sleep, and self-esteem. It has been found to be an effec-tive treatment when compared to no treatment. Also, exercise's antidepres-sant qualities continue after depressive symptoms abate, which makes it valuable as part of long-term management and relapse prevention. In gen-eral, exercise is safe and effective in the treatment of mild-to-moderate depression. Severely depressed patients are usually unable to exercise until partly recovered. Prematurely urging them to exercise adds to their feelings of failure and inadequacy. Prescribing exercise may be contraindicated for depressed patients with anorexia nervosa, who already may be compul-sively overexercising.

Sleep Hygiene

A disrupted sleep cycle is a common symptom of depression, and sleep deprivation is a recognized precipitant of depression. Poor sleep quality or quantity contributes to the higher incidence of postpartum depression, in rotating shift workers, in those with chronic pain, and in cases of substance abuse. Some patients have lifestyles entailing chronically poor sleep habits.

A review of the patient's sleep pattern and instruction on proper sleep hygiene is often very helpful. Simple information sheets can be provided including reminders to only be in bed when ready for sleep, to not read or watch television in bed for prolonged periods, to avoid drinking fluids before bed that may cause nocturnal urination, and to avoid stimulating substances in the late afternoon or evening. Failure to change poor sleep habits will undermine the effectiveness of therapies for depression and promote relapse.

Nutrition and Hydration

Though eating correctly and maintaining adequate hydration may seem obvious, they are frequently overlooked in the management of the depressed patient. Reduction in intake of food and fluids or overconsumption of junk food are often habits co-occurring with depressive symptoms. If malnutrition or dehydration are sustained or if the patient was already in a vulnerable state (e.g., chronically ill, elderly), secondary problems can occur, including alteration of medication metabolism and orthostasis secondary to dehydration. If prolonged, electrolyte derangement and vitamin deficiencies may occur. Some depressed patients may benefit from oral nutritional supplements. B vitamin supplementation has been studied in treatment-resistant depression with mixed results; a daily multivitamin cannot hurt and may help.

St. John's Wort and Other Alternative Medicine Therapies

St. John's wort, a common flowering plant (*Hypericum perforatum*), is widely sold in the United States as a dietary supplement. Many Americans now take this preparation for depressive symptoms even though the FDA does not evaluate its efficacy or purity because it is not considered a "medication." Hypericin, a naphthodianthrone, is considered the active ingredient. It is not known if hypericin crosses the blood-brain barrier, but in vitro, it inhibits the reuptake of the neurotransmitters serotonin, norepinephrine, and dopamine and binds to GABA receptors. The metabolism and excretion of hypericin is unknown at this time. In Germany, St. John's wort is licensed for the treatment of anxiety, depression, and insomnia, and, not surprisingly, most of the studies using hypericin for the treatment of depression come from Europe. The results are difficult to apply clinically because there is no consistent, reliable source for hypericin in the United States. As a result, studies that test hypericin have to make their own preparations. However, the available data suggest that hypericin is relatively safe and may be effective in the treatment of mild depression. Most experienced clinicians consider it ineffective for severe depression. However, St. John's wort is a potent inducer of cytochrome P450 enzymes (particularly CYP3A4) and P-glycoprotein. Its co-administration has resulted in decreased plasma concentrations for a number of drugs, including amitriptyline, cyclosporine, digoxin, indinavir, warfarin, alprazolam, simvastatin, and oral contraceptives.

St. John's wort should not be combined with SSRIs because of the risk of serotonin syndrome.

Patients may turn to a wide variety of other herbal or nutritional remedies purported to have antidepressant effects, such as gingko, kava kava, melatonin, megavitamin doses, DHEA, chromium, inositol, and S-adenosyl methionine. Full discussion is beyond the scope of this book, but these agents have even less evidence to support their usage. Clinicians are urged to carefully ask patients what they may be taking because of unrecognized risks for side effects and drug interactions.

Reduction of Psychoactive Substances

Patients frequently consume substances, in some cases as a form of self-treatment, that may precipitate or aggravate depressive symptoms or adversely affect antidepressant treatment.

Caffeine is probably the most widely used psychoactive substance (see Chapter 12). Many patients with depressive symptoms, particularly fatigue and decreased concentration, may self-medicate with caffeine. In addition to coffee, tea, caffeinated soda, and herbal beverages (e.g., yerba mate, guarana), caffeine may be consumed in over-the-counter (OTC) preparations for weight loss, headache, and staying awake. A few patients are especially sensitive to caffeine and experience side effects even at lower doses (e.g., 1-2 caffeinated drinks). When taken regularly in high quantities (e.g., more than 4 caffeinated drinks per day), caffeine may produce anxiety and interfere with sleep. A withdrawal syndrome characterized by irritability, depression, lethargy, headache, and decreased concentration may occur particularly in the late afternoon. Excessive consumption of caffeine interferes with the normalization of sleep that marks antidepressants' efficacy. Too much caffeine may also aggravate side effects (e.g., jitteriness, diarrhea, and insomnia) of antidepressants, especially SSRIs, SNRIs, and bupropion. Over-the-counter decongestants may cause side effects including jitteriness and sleeplessness on their own account, or they may interact with antidepressants causing side effects as well. Because OTC sympathomimetics are nonspecific adrenergic agonists, tachyphylaxis is common; some patients are addicted and use large quantities (e.g., nasal decongestant spray). Sedating antihistamines may aggravate the mental slowing of depression or sedation side effect of antidepressants. The preferred treatments for allergic upper respiratory symptoms in depressed patients are nonsedating antihistamines and nasal steroids. When a patient comes in during cold or allergy season with new side effects on a stable antidepressant regimen, a possible OTC drug reaction or interaction should be considered.

A wide variety of alternative medicine preparations have contained sympathomimetic compounds, primarily "natural" ephedrine (often identified as ephedra or ma huang). Like OTC sympathomimetics, such herbal supplements may cause poor sleep and jitteriness by interacting with medications or in their own right. This has become less common in the United

States since the FDA prohibited the sale of dietary supplements containing ephedrine alkaloids (e.g., ephedra) in February 2004, because such supplements present an unreasonable risk of illness or injury.

Alcohol is the quintessential form of self-treatment. In the short term, for some it causes a feeling of well-being and relaxation and helps initiate sleep. Yet because it is a CNS depressant, it eventuates in worsening depression. It ultimately erodes the quality and quantity of sleep by disrupting REM sleep, decreasing motivation and self-esteem, and contributing to poor nutrition. It is appropriate to urge cessation of all alcohol during the initial phases of treatment of depression. When the symptoms of depression have abated, cautious, limited resumption of alcohol can be considered. Advising no more than 1 drink per day is prudent.

Patients should be asked about any other psychoactive substance use. Chronic daily use of marijuana may be associated with depression, apathy, and decreased ability to concentrate. Even occasional usage should be discouraged in actively depressed patients. Cocaine and amphetamines cause the release of brain catecholamines. Repeated usage leads to a vicious cycle of catecholamine depletion with intense feelings of depression, resulting in increased abuse and then ultimately a "crash." There are often depressive withdrawal symptoms following cessation of regular use of cocaine or amphetamines.

Relaxation Techniques

Relaxation techniques like meditation, yoga, tai chi, and other mind-body therapies may be helpful in managing some of the anxiety symptoms associated with depression, and there are easy-to-learn forms adapted for general use. These practices, though simple, require effort and motivation on the patient's part. Depressed patients often lack energy and motivation, making relaxation techniques usually impractical in the moderately to severely depressed patient. However, in the mildly depressed patient with anxiety or in long-term treatment, relaxation techniques can be an important adjunct. Many psychotherapists, as well as physical and occupational therapists, are familiar with relaxation techniques and can teach them to patients; there are increasing numbers of nonmedical sources for them, too.

Religious Involvement

Isolation and disconnection from social support are often seen in depression. Depression occurs less often in people with religious involvement as opposed to those with no religious involvement. Recent studies have shown a decreased likelihood of depression in frequent church attendees. It is unclear what provides the protective value; social support, instillation of hope, a sense of life's meaning, acceptance of suffering, and other spiritual values are some of the possibilities that could explain religion's protective value. It appears that the cognition of an ordered world (e.g., faith and trust in God) offers some protective value for the psychological symptoms of depression but less for the somatic symptoms of depression. While a clinician cannot "prescribe" religion, a careful review of past religious involvement may uncover a potential avenue for support that could be reinvigorated with the clinician's encouragement. Sometimes depression is precipitated by a loss that challenges the patient's faith or causes spiritual alienation. Clergy or pastoral counselors can add meaningful help for depressed patients with these "psychoreligious" conflicts.

Patient Education and Support Groups

Many patients and their families can benefit from educational material, and the organizations listed in the Box 4-9 are good sources for printed and Web-based information. For those who wish for more in-depth information,

---

Box 4-9 National Organizations and Access Information

Depression Awareness, Recognition, and Treatment (D/ART) Program
National Institute of Mental Health
5600 Fishers Lane, Room 14C03
Parklawn Building, Rockville, MD 20857
800-421-4211
301-443-4140

Depression and Related Affective Disorders Association (DRADA)
8201 Greensboro Drive, Suite 300, McLean, VA 22102
703-610-9026
888-288-1104

Depressives Anonymous: Recovery from Depression
329 East 62nd Street, New York, NY 10021
212-689-2600

National Depressive and Manic-Depressive Association
730 North Franklin Street, Suite 501, Chicago, IL 60610
800-82-NDMDA
Fax: 312-642-7243

National Foundation for Depressive Illness, Inc.
PO Box 2257, New York, NY 10116
800-239-1265
http://www.depression.org

Mental Health Information Center
800-969-NMHA
Crisis Hotline: 800-273-TALK (800-273-8255)
TTY Line: 800-433-5959
http://www.nmha.org

there are a number of good books (see Box 4-10). Educational materials are useful adjuncts to treatment, but they are primarily effective in reinforcing information provided by the primary health providers and mental health professionals. Clinical research suggests that if the educational material is not supported by the health care providers, then there is little impact on patient behavior. Patient educational material should not replace patient-clinician dialogue, which remains one of the most powerful means of behavior change in patients.

Social isolation is a risk factor, a symptom, and a cause of depression. Steps taken to counter social isolation directly are helpful. This may be as simple as the clinician encouraging the depressed patient to have more contact with family, friends, and community. For patients with depression, as with other chronic medical illnesses, support groups can help by providing an opportunity to share experiences with others with the same condition. Clinicians should learn what resources are locally available. Box 4-9 lists national sources of information regarding mental health referral, support groups, and depression in general.

> **Box 4-10 Self-help Books on Depression**
>
> *Understanding Depression: What We Know and What You Can Do About It* by Raymond DePaulo Jr., et al. (New York: Wiley, 2005)
> *The Noonday Demon: An Atlas of Depression* by Andrew Solomon (New York: Simon and Schuster Trade, 2001)
> *Free Yourself from Depression* by Michael D. Yapko (Emmaus, PA: Rodale Press, 1992)

KEY POINTS

- Response rates to initial monotherapies for depression vary between 40% to 60%.
- Remission rates are lower (30%-50%) than response rates.
- Before initiating any treatment the general clinician should do the following:
  - Establish the diagnosis.
- Reviewing the longitudinal course of the symptoms is necessary to distinguish dysthymia from single-episode or recurrent major depression.
  - Clarify with the patient the target symptoms (i.e., the symptoms that are impacting the patient's functioning).
  - Carefully consider the patient's preference.
- Patient education at this point can mitigate against misinformation and lay the groundwork for reasonable expectations.
- Introduce psychotherapy early as an option, especially if chronic symptoms or acute stressors are present.

- In pharmacotherapy, using the full dosage of an antidepressant for an adequate period of time (6-12 weeks) is more important than the choice of a particular antidepressant.
- Initial follow-ups should be frequent, at least every 4 to 6 weeks (2 weeks is ideal). These can occur over the phone or with a non-MD. Education, response, and side effects are the focus of these contacts and are significantly correlated with improved outcomes for patients.
- Antidepressants should be continued for at least 9 months *after* full response or remission. This means most antidepressants are taken for at least 1 year.
- Long-term maintenance therapy should be considered when the chance of recurrence is high (i.e., multiple episodes, residual symptoms, chronic stressors, comorbid diseases).
- CBT has the greatest empirical evidence supporting its usage as a monotherapy for mild-to-moderate depression.

REFERENCES

1. Wang PS, Lane M, Olfson M, et al. Twelve-month use of mental health services in the United States: results from the national comorbidity survey replication. *Arch Gen Psychiatry.* 2005;62:629-640.

2. *Practice Guideline for the Treatment of Patients with Major Depressive Disorder.* 2nd ed. Washington, DC: American Psychiatric Association; 2000.

3. Kerr GW, McGuffie AC, Wilkie S. Tricyclic antidepressant overdose: a review. *Emerg Med J.* 2001;18(4):236-241.

4. CAST Investigators. Preliminary report: effect of encainide and flecainide on mortality in a randomized trial of arrhythmia suppression after myocardial infarction. The cardiac arrhythmia suppression trial. *N Engl J Med.* 1989; 321(6):406-412.

5. Rush AJ, Kraemer HC, Sackeim HA, et al. Report by the ACNP Task Force on response and remission in major depressive disorder. *Neuropsychopharmacology.* 2006;31:1841-1853.

6. Simon GE, Heiligenstein JH, Grothaus L, et al. Should anxiety and insomnia influence antidepressant selection: a randomized comparison of fluoxetine and imipramine. *J Clin Epidemiol.* 1998;59(2):49-55.

7. Clark MR, Chodynicki MP. Pain. In: Levenson JL, ed. *Essentials of Psychosomatic Medicine.* Washington, DC: American Psychiatric Publishing; 2007:451-492.

KEY REFERENCES

Boyer EW, Shannon M. The serotonin syndrome. *N Engl J Med.* 2005;352:1112-1120.

Butler AC, Chapman JE, Forman EM, et al. The empirical status of cognitive-behavioral therapy: a review of meta-analyses. *Clin Psychol Rev.* 2006;26:17-31.

Casacalenda N, Perry JC, Looper K. Remission in Major Depressive Disorder: a comparison of pharmacotherapy, psychotherapy, and control conditions. *Am J Psychiatry.* 2002;159:1354-1360.

Clark MR, Chodynicki MP. Pain. In: Levenson JL, ed., *American Psychiatric Publishing Textbook of Psychosomatic Medicine.* Washington, DC: American Psychiatric Publishing; 2005:827-870.

Coppen A, Bolander-Gouaille C. Treatment of depression: time to consider folic acid and vitamin B12. *J Psychopharmacol.* 2005;19:59-65.

DeRubeis RJ, Hollon SD, Amsterdam JD, et al. Cognitive therapy vs medications in the treatment of moderate to severe depression. *Arch Gen Psychiatry.* 2005;62(4):409-416.

Dunn AL, Trivedi MH, Kampert JB, Clark CG, Chambliss HO. Exercise treatment for depression: efficacy and dose response. *Am J Prev Med.* 2005;28:1-8.

Gregorian RS, Golden KA, Bahce A, et al. Antidepressant-induced sexual dysfunction. *Ann Pharmacother.* 2002;36:1577-1589.

Kessler RC, Berglund P, Demler O, et al. The epidemiology of major depressive disorder: results from the National Comorbidity Survey Replication (NCS-R). *JAMA.* 2003;289:3095-3105.

McKendree-Smith NL, Floyd M, Scogin FR. Self-administered treatments for depression: a review. *J Clin Psychol.* 2003;275-288.

Robinson MJ, Owen JA. Psychopharmacology. In: Levenson JL, ed. *The American Psychiatric Publishing Textbook of Psychosomatic Medicine.* Washington, DC: American Psychiatric Publishing; 2005:871-922.

Trivedi MH, Rush AJ, Wisniewski SR, et al. Evaluation of outcomes with citalopram for depression using measurement-based care in STAR*D: implications for clinical practice. *Am J Psychiatry.* 2006;163:28-40.

Treatment of Major Depression and Dysthymia: What to Do When the Initial Intervention Fails

The first treatment regimen for depression is frequently ineffective or inadequate. In fact, after an adequate initial trial of a single antidepressant, failure, *not* reaching remission (60%-70%), is twice as likely as success, remission (30%). When success is redefined as response, at least 50% reduction in symptoms, the "success" rate can climb to 40% to 60%. However, most patients do not find a 50% reduction of presenting symptoms to be a "success" (1).

In this chapter, we will review some of the recent results of the Sequenced Treatment Alternatives to Relieve Depression (STAR*D) trial, which was sponsored by the National Institute of Mental Health (NIMH). The STAR*D study is the largest prospective study of a sequential series of treatments for depression ever conducted. The study entered over 4000 eligible subjects at 41 sites in the United States, 18 of which were general medical settings. The results varied little between general medical and specialty mental health sites. In this chapter, we will highlight the results from STAR*D as we discuss different strategies for treating depression after the first attempt fails (2).

Treatment-Resistant Depression vs "Pseudoresistance"

As many as 40% of patients receiving antidepressant therapies may be considered "treatment resistant." However, "treatment resistance" may not represent a true state of treatment nonresponse; these "nonresponding" patients may instead have not received adequate treatment or have been misdiagnosed. A medical example is a patient who has a blood pressure of 135/98 after receiving 25 mg of hydrochlorothiazide (HCTZ) for 6 months. This patient's hypertension is not "treatment resistant"; rather, the treatment is inadequate. Likewise, a patient with depressive symptoms that are not resolving with 100 mg of sertraline is probably not treatment resistant but instead is undertreated. When a patient's depression is incorrectly labeled as "treatment-resistant depression," we refer to this as "pseudoresistance" (see Box 5-1).

We divide the causes of pseudoresistance into 2 groups: patient factors and clinician factors. The most common reasons for treatment failures are inadequate trials of antidepressants because of either too low of a dose of the antidepressant or too short a duration of treatment. Patients (and

---

Box 5-1 Pseudoresistance:
Associated Factors

Clinician Factors
- Inadequate dose of anti-depressant
- Too short a duration of treatment
- Incorrect diagnosis
  - Medical mimics
  - Comorbid conditions are not diagnosed (medical, psychiatric, and substance use)
  - Depressive subtype is misdiagnosed as *only* major depression
    - Psychotic Depression
    - Bipolar Disorders in a depressive episode
    - Premenstrual dysphoric disorder

Patient Factors
- Noncompliance
- Social comorbidity (e.g., poverty, abuse, job loss)
- Unusual pharmacokinetics (e.g., poor absorption, rapid metabolism)

---

clinicians) become impatient or have unrealistic expectations for the time it takes for symptoms to remit and subsequently change agents before titrating up to a full dosage or waiting long enough for results. The need for adequate time for treatment was highlighted in the initial treatment step of STAR*D with citalopram (monotherapy), where the mean time for the subjects who achieved *remission* (i.e., essentially no symptoms) was 12 weeks and where only 56% of the subjects who had a *response* (i.e., a 50% reduction in symptoms) did not do so until 8 weeks or later (2). Waiting to see if an agent will be effective is very hard to do with depressed patients in large measure because patients are continuing to suffer. Frequent contact with patients early in treatment serves not only to monitor symptoms but also to support the patient through the difficult time of waiting and to bolster adherence.

When patients' depressive symptoms do not abate despite treatment trials of adequate dose and duration, the diagnosis of depression should be reconsidered. Medical, psychiatric, and substance use disorders are frequently comorbid and can cause symptoms that mimic depression (discussed in Chapter 3).

Patient noncompliance is another significant cause of nonresponse. Patients frequently alter their medication regimens by taking their medications only on days they feel bad or at a reduced dosage. A large fraction of antidepressant prescriptions are not refilled by patients, often without admitting this to their clinicians. Problems of adherence are not unique to psychiatric disorders and should be familiar to clinicians, particularly in the treatment of chronic medical disorders (e.g., diabetes, hypertension, hypercholesterolemia). Directly discussing compliance with the patient is usually sufficient, but sometimes measuring serum levels of the agent can detect poor compliance or, in rare cases, unusual metabolism (e.g., rapid metabolism or poor absorption). Obtaining a collateral history from the patient's past records or a companion is also helpful when assessing compliance.

After pseudoresistance has been ruled out, true treatment-resistant depression is considered. Thase and Rush (1997) have devised a multistage

---

Box 5-2 Classification of Treatment-Resistant Depression

Stage 0: No single adequate trial of medication
Stage 1: No response to an adequate trial of one medication
Stage 2: Failure to respond to 2 different adequate monotherapy trials of
        medications from different classes
Stage 3: Stage 2 plus failure to respond to first augmentation strategy
Stage 4: Stage 3 plus failure to respond to a second augmentation strategy
Stage 5: Stage 4 plus failure to respond to electroconvulsive therapy

---

system for classifying depressions that are truly resistant to treatment (see Box 5-2). They take into account that treatment resistance is a relative concept as opposed to an absolute. They define treatment resistance by the treatment strategies that have failed. This classification system is useful when reviewing a patient's past treatment experiences (3).

■ Switching vs Adding Another Agent (Augmentation and Dual Therapy)

As noted in the previous section, waiting for a response, let alone remission, is challenging—especially when most of the time a full response will not occur and, when it does, it usually takes a long time (e.g., 6-8 weeks). If a patient has not had an adequate response to an adequate trial, the main options are either switching to a different antidepressant or adding a second drug (see Figure 5-1). Switching is often chosen if there has been little or no response or severe side effects with the initial antidepressant. An additional agent (called "dual therapy" when the second drug is another antidepressant and "augmentation" when it is from a different drug family) is often added if some response, but not remission, occurred. The difference between augmentation and dual therapy is subtle but important. Augmentation implies that the initial agent has the primary antidepressant effect and the additional agent facilitates the initial agent's antidepressant function (e.g., lithium, buspirone, and T3). In dual therapy, the second agent is another antidepressant; it is as though the patient is receiving 2 monotherapies. Examples of dual therapies include an SSRI plus bupropion, an SSRI plus trazodone, and an SNRI plus mirtazapine. On the following pages, we will first review some additional important findings from the STAR*D study, then review switching antidepressants and using combination strategies (including psychotherapy) in detail.

STAR*D confirmed that about one-third of patients achieve remission with initial single antidepressant treatment (Step 1) and that remission rates decline with successive treatment trials. Higher remission rates during the initial trial were seen in patients who were female, Caucasian, employed, or had higher levels of education and income. Alternatively, patients who

Depression Treatment Strategy: Switch vs Augment

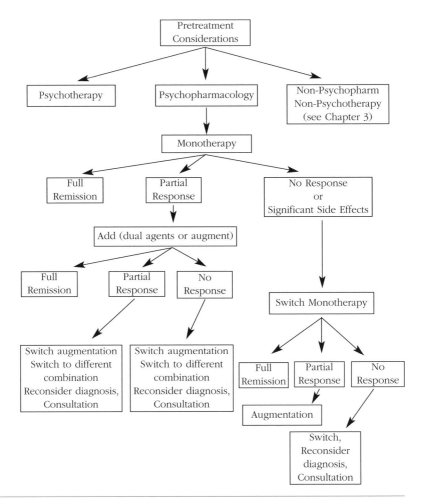

Figure 5-1

required more treatments were more severely depressed and had more concurrent psychiatric and medical disorders.

STAR*D results showed essentially no difference in remission rates (about 25%) regardless of the agent or class of drug. Specifically, switching to bupropion or venlafaxine were no different than switching to sertraline, which is another SSRI like citalopram. These results strongly suggest that focusing on an antidepressant's effect on a particular neurotransmitter system is less important than optimizing dosage for an adequate period of time (see Chapter 4 for more on particular monotherapies).

Switching Antidepressants

The decision of which antidepressant to switch to does not occur in a vacuum. The experience of the first trial, for better or worse, informs the switch decision. For example, though STAR*D found little difference between the switch scenarios from citalopram to bupropion (different drug classes) and from citalopram to sertraline (same drug class), many patients (and some clinicians) prefer not to use agents from the same class when switching. Further clarifying the patient's target symptoms and repeating the other pretreatment considerations outlined in Chapter 4 will help guide the choice of the second antidepressant to try.

One important pretreatment consideration to revisit is past treatment outcomes. When switching to another agent, it is important to remember that the "new" agent may not be "new" to the patient. However, it is worthwhile to consider *why* past treatment may have failed before rejecting the idea of switching to that agent. Frequently, patients report having "failed" treatment with a particular agent, when in fact the agent was either dosed improperly or inadequately. For example, a patient may have experienced agitation and tremor in the past with bupropion and subsequently stopped it after 4 days. With further clarification, the patient reports that the starting dose was 300 mg in the morning and that he or she regularly consumed 4 to 6 cups of coffee each morning. The combination of the high starting dose of bupropion with significant caffeine consumption produced a predictable outcome. In this example, the patient could be instructed to reduce caffeine consumption before starting at a lower initial dosage of bupropion (e.g., 100 mg).

There is little evidence to guide clinicians on the best way to stop one agent and start another. Three options exist: (1) stop one agent completely and immediately start the next; (2) taper the initial agent's dosage down, while simultaneously titrating the new agent's dosage up (i.e., cross taper); and (3) taper the initial agent's dosage gradually down and stop completely (i.e., wash out) before starting the new agent and gradually titrating its dosage up. The respective classes, half-lives, and interactions of the agents suggest which option to use.

Generally, switching agents from the same class (e.g., from one SSRI to another) can be accomplished using the first strategy of stopping one completely and immediately starting another. The major caveat involves the half-life of the initial agent. Long half-life antidepressants like fluoxetine essentially self-taper and can be stopped completely without a taper. However, long half-life agents can magnify the second agent's effect by interfering with the new agent's metabolism in the liver or combining its residual serotoninergic effects with the new agent's. Either situation can result in a greater incidence of side effects or, very rarely, in extreme cases of serotonin syndrome. Starting the second agent at a low dose 2 or 3 days after stopping fluoxetine and subsequently titrating it up slowly works best.

When the first agent has a very short half-life or when switching between classes of antidepressants, using the second switching option of cross tapering is recommended. (Switching to an MAOI is a significant exception that is discussed in the next paragraph.) Antidepressants with short half-lives and no (or few) active metabolites (e.g., paroxetine, immediate-release venlafaxine) are more likely to cause a discontinuation syndrome and should be tapered. Remember that all antidepressants can cause discontinuation syndrome when abruptly stopped (see Chapter 4).

Tapering the first agent completely off and allowing time for it to wash out before the new agent is started is primarily reserved for situations where potentially dangerous interactions between the 2 agents exist (e.g., hypertensive crisis with MAOIs, serotonin syndrome). When switching to an MAOI, different wash out periods are required depending on the antidepressant and its class. SSRIs and TCAs typically require at least 2 weeks, but fluoxetine requires 5 weeks because of the long half-life of its active metabolite norfluoxetine. These examples further support the recommendation of leaving treatment with MAOIs to psychiatrists.

Combination Strategies (Augmentation and Dual Therapy)

Combination strategies (as opposed to switching strategies) are typically considered when there is a partial response to the initial monotherapy but remission of symptoms is not attained. This occurs when there is a plateauing of the response despite a maximum dose or when significant side effects occur that prevent further dose increases. Combination strategies have been typically studied separately but rarely comparatively. The combinations studied in STAR*D include an SSRI plus buspirone, an SSRI plus bupropion, venlafaxine plus mirtazapine, mirtazapine plus lithium or T3, and nortriptyline plus lithium or T3. Trazodone and stimulants will also be reviewed. Other combination treatments such as an antidepressant plus either an antipsychotic or a mood stabilizer (except lithium) are beyond the scope of this book and are discussed elsewhere (see References).

■ Psychotherapy Combination

There is a large database that describes and supports the combination of psychotherapy with antidepressants. Psychotherapy should be considered early in treatment because it can be used in a broad range of situations; it has several forms, and the side-effect burden is very low. Psychotherapy (e.g., cognitive behavioral therapy [CBT]) used as a monotherapy for the treatment of depression is reviewed in depth in Chapter 4. The discussion here will pick up with the use of psychotherapy in combination with medications.

The combination of psychotherapy with medication is particularly potent for patients who experience chronic or recurrent major depression in both acute and maintenance phases of treatment. For example, a patient with chronic fatigue secondary to depression may have a hard time increasing activity after successful antidepressant treatment because he or she still believes and behaves as though he or she is depressed and therefore fatigued. Another patient may experience relief in depressive symptoms affecting energy, sleep, and concentration but still have low self-esteem or problems with interpersonal relationships. These residual beliefs and behaviors are directly addressed in psychotherapy. In a large clinical trial, Keller et al (2000) randomly assigned adults with chronic depression (i.e., major depression for 2 years or longer) to receive an antidepressant (nefazodone) alone, CBT alone, or a combination of both therapies. The overall response rate of those who attended at least 1 session (662 of 681) was 48% in the nefazodone group and in the psychotherapy group compared with 73% in the combined treatment group. Of the 519 subjects who completed the study, the response rates were even higher: the nefazodone group had a 55% response rate, the psychotherapy group had a 52% response rate, and the group who received the combination of both had an 85% response rate. The medication produced effects more rapidly than did CBT, but by week 12 the efficacy of the 2 approaches was similar. The combined treatment appeared to have an additive effect that became evident between weeks 4 and 5 and was sustained to the end of the 12-week trial (4).

Combining CBT and pharmacotherapy appears particularly effective in preventing relapse or recurrence during the period of highest risk, that is, in the first 6 months following remission or recovery. In another study, 187 subjects with recurrent depression who had reached remission with various pharmacotherapies were randomly assigned to continue their pharmacotherapy with and without CBT. They were assessed for relapse or recurrence for 2 years. By combining CBT with pharmacotherapy, a significant protective effect was experienced, which only intensified with the number of previous depressive episodes. For patients with 5 or more previous episodes (41% of the sample), CBT combined with pharmacotherapy reduced relapse and recurrence rates from 72% to 46% over 2 years (5).

■ Pharmacotherapy Combinations

The following agents are commonly added to the initial antidepressant when it fails to provide remission of the patient's depressive symptoms (see Chapter 4 for a detailed discussion of these antidepressants and major side effects).

Tri-iodothyromine (T-3) and Lithium Augmentation

T-3 and lithium were some of the first agents studied for augmentation of antidepressant treatment. Most of the early studies involved augmenting

TCAs. The currently available evidence supports using these agents more often than they are being used. A meta-analysis of T-3 augmentation showed a consistently positive effect when compared to adding a placebo, but the degree of the positive effect is hard to determine because mostly response (rather than remission) was measured. A large meta-analysis of lithium augmentation showed a response rate of 45% compared to a rate with placebo of 18% (6). STAR*D compared T-3 and lithium augmentation of nortriptyline or mirtazapine after 2 prior treatment failures. The remission rates were 24.7% (T-3) and 15.9% (lithium), but the number of subjects was too small for statistical comparison. There was a significantly higher dropout rate with lithium than T-3 (7). The Texas Medication Algorithm Project (TMAP) currently recommends lithium augmentation before switching or adding another antidepressant.

Lithium augmentation is usually initiated at 300 mg/day and may be increased to 300 mg 2 to 3 times a day; T-3 is started at 25 mcg and can be increased to 50 mcg/day. Thyroid function is usually not greatly affected by the low dose of T-3, but a thyroid-simulating hormone (TSH) should be checked to avoid overly suppressing it. Lithium can cause hypothyroidism, so thyroid function should be followed (see Chapter 6 for more on lithium).

Buspirone

Buspirone (BuSpar) by itself is not an effective treatment for major depression, but it has shown some value in augmentation. Buspirone is most often used with SSRIs and SNRIs but can also be used with TCAs. Patients with residual symptoms of anxiety, restlessness, or irritability are particularly good candidates for buspirone augmentation. Buspirone is taken 2 to 3 times a day. The 15 mg pills are scored in halves and thirds, allowing slow titration and exact dosing. The starting dose is 15 mg/day in divided doses (5 mg 3 times a day or 7.5 mg 2 times a day), which is titrated up to 30 mg/day within 1 to 3 weeks. The maximum dose is 60 to 90 mg/day, though many patients respond at lower doses. The major dose-limiting side effects are dizziness, nausea, and sedation.

Adding Bupropion

Bupropion (Wellbutrin) is often combined with SSRIs and SNRIs but can be combined with TCAs or mirtazapine. Bupropion is a stimulating antidepressant and is a good choice for many patients who have residual symptoms of fatigue, lethargy, and apathy. It is also a good choice for augmentation if the first agent has caused sexual dysfunction. The evidence is mixed as to whether or not sexual dysfunction can be reversed by bupropion, but its addition may allow a reduction of the initial antidepressant dosage, and, in some cases, it may completely replace the initial agent. The sustained-release form is most commonly used with a starting dose of 100 mg. The dosage can be titrated up to maximum doses slowly if needed.

Overactivation, jitteriness, and occasionally tremors are side effects that can occur, especially at higher doses.

Adding a TCA

Adding a TCA should be considered in patients with residual insomnia, agitation, chronic pain, anxiety, or chronic severe depressive symptoms. Though amitriptyline is appealing when neuropathic pain is present, its side-effect burden (primarily anticholinergic) limits its usage. When a TCA is considered, we suggest using a secondary amine, particularly nortriptyline (amitriptyline's metabolite), starting at 25 mg at bedtime and gradually increasing the dose. Keep in mind that lower doses should be used when augmenting fluoxetine and paroxetine because they inhibit TCA metabolism and therefore increase TCA blood levels, which can be measured if needed.

Adding Trazodone

The addition of trazodone to another antidepressant is a common strategy, either for augmentation or to target a specific symptom (e.g., insomnia). Patients with either SSRI-induced insomnia or a residual depression-related sleep disturbance are especially responsive to lower doses of trazodone. The typical dose is between 25 mg and 100 mg at bedtime, but some patients need and tolerate much higher doses.

Adding Mirtazapine

In addition to being an effective monotherapy, mirtazapine (Remeron) is often used in combination with SSRIs, SNRIs, and bupropion. Its combination with a TCA would amplify their similar side-effect profiles (e.g., sedation, weight gain). The addition of mirtazapine is typically considered when symptoms of insomnia or decreased appetite persist, adding 15 mg at bedtime and increasing slowly if necessary. If morning drowsiness occurs, move the dosing to earlier in the evening (i.e., before 10:00 PM).

■ Stimulants

The stimulants D-amphetamine (Dexedrine) and methylphenidate (Ritalin) were released in the United States in 1937 and 1954, respectively. Since their release, they have been used to treat depression. Stimulants can be used as a monotherapy, as an initial treatment until an antidepressant starts to have its effects, and in combination with long-term use of an antidepressant. The following section discusses each of the clinical situations where a stimulant may be helpful.

Stimulants in Debilitated Patients

Stimulants have several different applications for the medically ill. Severely debilitated patients (especially those in the hospital) in early recovery from acute illness (e.g., stroke) who are apathetic, have psychomotor retardation, are not eating, or are not participating in care (e.g., physical therapy, occupational therapy) may respond well to a short course of a stimulant. The initiation of a low dose of methylphenidate (e.g., 2.5-10 mg) in the early morning (i.e., 8:00 AM) and at noon can positively affect eating and motivation to participate in care. If these symptoms are believed to represent major depression, then either an antidepressant can be added and the stimulant stopped, or, in some cases, the stimulant can be continued as a monotherapy.

Patients with chronic medical illnesses (e.g., cancer, HIV, multiple sclerosis) involving chronic pain, fatigue, or diminished concentration can often be managed with a stimulant as a monotherapy. Predictably rapid onset of action and few drug-drug interactions make stimulants a particularly useful option. The elderly who are medically frail may be particularly good candidates for stimulants for the reasons outlined previously.

There are 2 significant caveats with stimulant use. Some patients become delirious with stimulants, especially when the dose is titrated up. It is unusual to see delirium at low doses of methylphenidate (e.g., 2.5-5.0 mg), but it can occur. The other potential problems are increased heart rate and blood pressure. Scheduled close observation and vital signs checks after the initial doses and after dose changes will detect problems early. Heart rate and blood pressure are usually unaffected by low doses of stimulants. These drugs have short half-lives, so any problems are short-lived.

Stimulant Use in Medically Ill Patients Needing a Quick Response

Medically ill patients (not necessarily debilitated) who are suffering from major depression and cannot wait 6 to 8 weeks for a response from a traditional antidepressant are good candidates for stimulant therapy. Initiating a stimulant can produce significant benefits in days. This strategy provides symptom relief until a traditional antidepressant can take effect. Like in the previous example, methylphenidate (Ritalin) is used in a single morning dose or in morning and afternoon doses. Methylphenidate at 2.5 to 5 mg at 8:00 AM and at noon is a typical start. If no response is noted within 2 days, the dose can be increased every 1 to 2 days by 10 mg, usually not exceeding a total dose of 40 mg per day. Once a response is seen, the clinician should monitor for length of response. Many patients only require a single morning dose because the effect lasts into the afternoon. After several weeks, the stimulant is tapered down because the antidepressant should be at adequate levels to have independent antidepressant effects. Stimulants are sometimes avoided in patients who have prominent anorexia and weight loss. If the decreased appetite or motivation to eat is related to the depression and apathy, then the stimulant will often actually improve the patient's eating. In most patients, stimulants at low doses do not cause anorexia. Given their relative safety and quick onset of action, a trial of stimulants should be considered earlier as opposed to later in the recovery of medically ill, deconditioned, depressed patients. Patients in palliative care are also good candidates for stimulants as the primary or sole treatment for depression because they benefit from the quick onset of action.

Adding a Stimulant to an Antidepressant

Clinicians should consider adding a stimulant to an antidepressant in patients who have residual depressive symptoms of fatigue, apathy, lethargy, and poor concentration. Short acting agents (e.g., methylphenidate, D-amphetamine, or generic Adderall) are used initially. After the dose is determined, the short-acting agent may be switched to a sustained-release form of the agent, which has the advantage of less frequent dosing, less abrupt effects, and less likelihood of abuse. Most times the stimulant is tapered after full remission, but some patients require long-term stimulant augmentation to maintain full remission. A psychiatric consultation is recommended if stimulant augmentation is needed.

■ Electroconvulsive Therapy

Electroconvulsive therapy (ECT) is an important consideration in the treatment of severe depression in which rapid reduction of symptoms is imperative, such as in cases of severe malnutrition, active suicidal intent, psychosis, catatonia, and pregnancy. ECT is also the most effective therapy for severe treatment-resistant depression. It is the seizure induced by ECT that is therapeutic, not the electrical impulse itself. ECT has been safely used in depressed patients with a wide variety of comorbid medical illnesses. The cardiac response immediately after ECT includes a sympathetically mediated increase in heart rate and blood pressure, followed by a vagally mediated bradycardia. Intracranial pressure increases with the seizure, so mass-occupying lesions or other reasons for increased intracranial pressure are relative contraindications to ECT. Anterograde amnesia frequently occurs during the course of ECT treatments; the amnesia gradually fades over a number of weeks. In a small minority of patients, persistent memory deficits occur.

Despite its well-documented safety and efficacy, ECT carries a significant stigma, and, in some states, there are additional regulations governing its usage. The roots of the stigma to ECT are in its early usage when it was applied without anesthesia and paralytic agents. During this early period, ECT was also overused in part because of the lack of pharmacological treatments. The book-turned-movie *One Flew over the Cuckoo's Nest* also contributed to the public's negative and inaccurate images of ECT. Since that time, diagnostic indications have been refined, and vast improvements in anesthesia and the stimulus parameters have occurred. Yet misinformation and, in some cases, unwarranted restriction of usage continue. The general clinician may be asked to advise patients and families after a recommendation for ECT has been given by a psychiatrist. The following are important things to review with patients who may receive ECT:

■ ECT is safe and efficacious. The death rate from ECT is <1/10,000 and is related to the anesthesia, not the ECT itself.
■ ECT is the electrical induction of generalized seizures for therapeutic purposes.
■ There are no absolute contraindications to ECT; it can be safely used in medically ill patients. The major risks involve anesthesia.
■ The normal course of ECT treatment is 6 to 12 treatments given at a rate of 2 to 3 per week.

■ Transcranial Magnetic Stimulation

In transcranial magnetic stimulation (TMS), a magnetic stimulus is used to induce a seizure instead of an electrical stimulus as in ECT. Though the extent of its efficacy and its role in the treatment of depression has not yet been established, the hope is that TMS will have less side effects and greater acceptance than ECT. However, a recent randomized controlled trial of TMS vs ECT found that TMS was not as effective as ECT, and ECT was substantially more effective for the short-term treatment of depression (8).

■ Vagal Nerve Stimulation

Vagal nerve stimulation (VNS) uses an implanted stimulator to send impulses along the left vagus nerve. It was approved in 1997 for the treatment of partial complex seizures, and in 2005 the FDA approved VNS for refractory depression. An open-label study of 59 subjects with severe treatment-resistant depression reported remission rates of 15% after 3 months, 27% after 1 year, and 22% after 2 years of medications and adjunctive VNS (9). However, a more recent controlled double-blind trial of VNS for depression failed to demonstrate statistical improvement over a sham treatment after a 10-week course of treatment (8). The results from the long-term phase of this trial have not yet been published.

KEY POINTS

- Only 30% to 40% of initial treatments for depression provide full remission.
- STAR*D was the first large study to look at serial switching vs combination therapies in the treatment of depression.
- Look for "pseudoresistance" when assessing past episodes and treatment responses.
- Response, let alone remission, may not occur until 6 to 8 weeks after the initiation of treatment.
- Psychotherapy, particularly CBT, is effective in combination with antidepressants in achieving remission in patients with chronic and recurrent depression.
- CBT combined with medications in maintenance-phase treatment is associated with a significant reduction in relapse and recurrence rates.
- ECT is safe and efficacious in the treatment of severe depression.

REFERENCES

1. Rush AJ, Kraemer HC, Sackeim HA, et al. Report by the ACNP Task Force on response and remission in major depressive disorder. *Neuropsychopharmacology.* 2006;31:1841-1853.

2. Trivedi MH, Rush AJ, Wisniewski SR, et al. Evaluation of outcomes with citalopram for depression using measurement-based care in STAR*D: implications for clinical practice. *Am J Psychiatry.* 2006;163:28-40.

3. Thase ME, Rush AJ. When at first you don't succeed: sequential strategies for antidepressant nonresponders. *J Clin Psychiatry.* 1997;58:23-29.

4. Keller MB, McCullough JP, Klein DN, et al. A comparison of nefazodone, the cognitive behavioral-analysis system of psychotherapy and their combination for the treatment of chronic depression. *N Engl J Med.* 2000;342:1462-1470.

5. Bockting CL, Schene AH, Spinhoven P, et al. Preventing relapse/recurrence in recurrent depression with cognitive therapy: a randomized controlled trial. *J Consult Clin Psychol.* 2005;73:647-657.

6. Aronson R, Offman HJ, Joffe RT, et al. Triiodothyronine augmentation in the treatment of refractory depression: a meta-analysis. *Arch Gen Psychiatry.* 1996;53:842-848.

7. Nierenberg AA, Fava M, Trivedi MH, et al. A comparison of lithium and T(3) augmentation following two failed medication treatments for depression: a STAR*D report. *Am J Psychiatry.* 2006;163:1519-1530.

8. Eranti S, Mogg A, Pluck G, Landau S, et al. A randomized, controlled trial with 6-month follow-up of repetitive transcranial magnetic stimulation and electroconvulsive therapy for severe depression. *Am J Psychiatry.* 2007;164:73-81.

9. Nahas Z, Marangell LB, Husain MM, et al. Two-year outcome of vagus nerve stimulation (VNS) for treatment of major depressive episodes. *J Clin Psychiatry.* 2005;66(9):1097-1104.

KEY REFERENCES

Evans DL, Charney DS, Lewis L, et al. Mood disorders in the medically ill: scientific review and recommendations. *Biol Psychiatry.* 2005;58:175-189.

Kornstein S, Schneider R. Clinical features of treatment-resistant depression. *J Clin Psychiatry.* 2001;62:18-25.

Nahas Z, Burns C, Foust MJ, Short B, Herbsman T, George MS. Vagus nerve stimulation (VNS) for depression: what do we know now and what should be done next? *Curr Psychiatry Rep.* 2006;8:445-451.

Pagnin D, de Queiroz V, Pini S, Cassano GB. Efficacy of ECT in depression: a meta-analytic review. *J ECT.* 2004;20:13-20.

Practice Guideline for the Treatment of Patients With Major Depressive Disorder. 2nd ed. Washington, DC: American Psychiatric Association; 2000.

Bipolar Disorders

▪ Bipolar Disorders and the General Clinician

Bipolar disorders, arguably the most complex of the mood disorders, are difficult to treat, are easy to miss, cause great functional impairment, and have increased mortality rates. This is of particular concern because bipolar disorders are so common, with a combined 12-month prevalence of about 1% of the population. As many as one-third to two-thirds of patients with bipolar disorders do not receive appropriate treatment. This is due in part to underrecognition of hypomania and subsequent misdiagnosis, both in the specialty mental health and primary care sectors. There is an average delay of 7.5 to 10 years from the onset of symptoms until correct diagnosis. As many as 40% of psychiatric inpatients admitted with the diagnosis of unipolar depression may later be reclassified as bipolar type I after the clinician notes a previously unrecognized manic episode. Delayed diagnosis is a serious problem with potentially tragic consequences, as suicide is extremely common in persons with bipolar disorders. Suicide rates average approximately 1% annually, or perhaps 60 times higher than the general population rate of 0.015% annually.

Although bipolar disorders include episodes of dysphoric depressed mood—like the disorders reviewed in Chapters 3, 4, and 5—bipolar disorders also include mood symptoms that are not "depressive" (e.g., hypomania, mania, psychosis). The different states or phases of bipolar disorders (e.g., depressive, manic, mixed episodes) have different symptoms that are present in one phase but not another. This is complicated clinically because bipolar disorders are defined by several dissimilar episodes; a current episode may be depressive and appear to be major depression (i.e., unipolar depression) but in fact represent bipolar depression because a prior episode of mania or hypomania has occurred.

The general clinician's responsibilities include recognizing when "depression" is not just major depression (i.e. unipolar depression) but a phase of bipolar disorder and recognizing when symptoms like irritability and impulsivity are not isolated symptoms but rather manifestations of bipolar disorder (i.e., hypomania, mania). The "essentials" required to distinguish between mood disorders include understanding the signs and symptoms of mania and hypomania and how they manifest in bipolar disorders, recognizing "mimics" of bipolar disorders, and knowing the criteria for the bipolar diagnoses. The remainder of the chapter is dedicated to treatment

Table 6-1 Bipolar Disorders

Bipolar I	Mania
Bipolar II	Hypomania + Major Depression
Cyclothymia	Hypomania + Dysthymia

strategies for bipolar disorders (see Table 6-1). Discussion of acute mania and its treatment are beyond the scope of this text because acute mania requires urgent psychiatric inpatient care.

■ Essential Concepts and Terms

Bipolar I

Bipolar I is defined as one or more episodes of mania, but typically both depressive and manic episodes occur in the course of bipolar I. On average, a patient will have 3 episodes of depression before having a recognized episode of mania. It is confusing that the definition of bipolar I does not include depressive episodes when depressive episodes are common clinically. The reason for this is that mania uniquely distinguishes bipolar I from other psychiatric disorders. Also, bipolar I may, though infrequently, present with a manic episode (i.e., no prior depressive episodes) or, rarely, only have manic episodes. This narrow definition allows for the inclusion of both common and uncommon presentations.

Bipolar II

Bipolar II is defined as major depression and hypomania. Unlike bipolar I, the manic-like symptoms (i.e., hypomania) in bipolar II are not significant enough to distinguish this disorder from others without the inclusion of major depression. Like bipolar I, bipolar II usually has onset with an episode of major depression; some estimate that 33% to 55% of all presenting major depressions actually represent a depressive episode of a bipolar disorder rather than unipolar depression. Distinguishing unipolar from bipolar depressive episodes is exceedingly important because the treatment approaches are very different, as we will see. Table 6-2 offers some of the main differences between unipolar and bipolar depressions.

Cyclothymia

Cyclothymia represents dysthymia with a history of hypomania. Relative to bipolar I and II, cyclothymia is less severe, but it is still associated with significant impairment. When followed longitudinally, almost one-third of

Table 6-2 Comparison of Bipolar Depression and Unipolar Depression

	Bipolar Depression	Unipolar Depression
Sex ratio	Equal	Women > men
Age at onset	Teens, 20s, and 30s	30s, 40s, 50s
Postpartum episodes	More common	Less common
Onset of episode	Often abrupt	More insidious
Number of episodes	Numerous	Fewer
Psychomotor activity	Retardation > agitation	Agitation > retardation
Sleep	Hypersomnia > insomnia	Insomnia > hypersomnia
Family history	More common	Less common

Case Study

A 46-year-old woman was managed as an outpatient for 8 years with the diagnosis of recurrent major depression and social phobia. Her frequent symptoms of excess sleep, fatigue, and agitation were believed to be due to unipolar depression and an anxiety disorder. These symptoms were not recognized as part of a bipolar disorder until she was admitted to a psychiatric unit when she became agitated, psychotic, and suicidal after aggressive treatment with antidepressants. When bipolar disorder was explained to the patient she said, "This is what I have been trying to describe to you for years!"

people with cyclothymia will develop either bipolar I or II. Most of the discussion in this chapter is about bipolar I and II.

Mania and Hypomania

Appreciating the spectrum of mania-like symptoms in hypomania and mania is key to understanding bipolar disorders. The major distinctions used to differentiate mania from hypomania from "normal" mood are severity and duration of symptoms. Mania exists at the extreme end of symptom severity. It requires at least 7 days of severe symptoms, often including psychosis and suicidality as part of its presentation. Given its extreme nature, it is most easily defined and recognized as bipolar I. Hypomania, on the other hand, is less severe, involves less patient dysfunction, and requires a shorter duration of at least 4 days. For these reasons it is much harder to measure and therefore harder to study. To help remember the components involved with hypomania and mania, Dr William Falk at Massachusetts General Hospital developed the mnemonic DIGFAST:

Distractibility
Insomnia
Grandiosity
Flight of ideas
Activity
Speech
Thoughtlessness

Distractibility in mania manifests as the individual initiating multiple tasks and finishing none. People with mania "feel" as though they are accomplishing a lot, even though they clearly are not.

Insomnia is the decreased need or desire for sleep in mania. The next day, the person is typically not tired and may even have more energy.

Grandiosity is an inflated and unrealistic self-esteem. It need not involve delusions, but it may.

Flight of ideas is the subjective experience of racing thoughts. The clinician may experience it as not being able to follow the associations within the conversation with the manic patient.

Activity refers to the goal-directed behavior that manic people may exhibit. This can manifest as excessive focus and preoccupation with a work project or social activity. The manic individual feels unable (and often unwilling) to stop.

Speech refers to the pressured speech that can occur. In cases of pressured speech, it seems as though the patient cannot speak fast enough to keep up with his or her thoughts. In contrast, merely rapid speech is fast but generally trackable.

Thoughtlessness is also referred to as risk-taking behaviors. When risk-taking is associated with goal-directed activities, it can pose a problem because the patient disregards negative consequences. Examples of the combination include shopping and spending thousands of dollars, excessively seeking sexual encounters, or "partying" for days at a time.

Mania can be defined as either a euphoric state with 3 DIGFAST symptoms or a state of significant irritability with 4 DIGFAST symptoms. Whether the state is seen as euphoric or irritable, the definition of mania always includes significant dysfunction that lasts at least 7 days and hypomania that lasts at least 4 days. The time components in the definitions are arbitrary minimums that the DSM-IV established for research purposes; hypomania typically lasts at least 4 days but can last for weeks, and mania usually lasts longer (without treatment).

Mixed States

In addition to the purer, "polar" states of depressive or hypomanic and manic episodes, there are mixed states or episodes where criteria for both major depression and mania are met simultaneously. More commonly, however, people with bipolar disorders have depressive episodes with a few intermixed symptoms of mania. Recognizing a mixed state is important because of its high correlation with bipolar II. In one recent study, researchers found a major depressive episode with 2 manic symptoms in 71.8% of bipolar II patients and in 41.5% of unipolar patients. When the researchers defined "mixed state" as major depression plus 3 manic-like symptoms, the prevalence of bipolar II dropped to 46.6%, but the prevalence of unipolar depression dropped more dramatically to 7.6%. The treatment implications of this are significant; we review them in the section titled Treatment.

Cycling and Rapid Cycling

"Cycling" refers to the movement over time between episodes (i.e., depression, hypomania, mania, mixed). Classically, the word "bipolar" derives its meaning from the 2 "poles," mania and depression. Patients frequently refer to cycling as "mood swings." Though the term "mood swings" is descriptively apt, it is nonspecific and can represent many other conditions (see Mimics later in this chapter). The DSM-IV uses "polarity" to distinguish unipolar from bipolar depressions, but earlier researchers defined "manic-depression" by the high number of episodes of mood disturbance irrespective of "polarity." These early researchers based their view on the observation that the greater the number of episodes of disturbed mood, the greater the likelihood of bipolar disorder. This is helpful clinically because it is usually easier to count the episodes rather than define each one as depression, hypomania, mania, or a mixed episode. This is particularly true when viewing the episodes retrospectively through the patient's eyes.

Cycling is characterized along 3 dimensions: frequency (i.e., number of episodes/time), time between episodes (i.e., euthymia vs switching), and duration of the episode before switching. Each of these has implications for prognosis and resistance to treatment.

Per the DSM-IV, rapid cycling specifies a bipolar disorder with at least 4 episodes of mood disturbance in 12 months; this strict definition has the episodes separated by periods of normal mood, or euthymia. This tight definition of rapid cycling is useful when studying the phenomenon, but clinically it is much more likely for one episode to switch to another with no time interval between. This is referred to as "switching," or biphasic cycling. The terms ultrarapid cycling or multiphasic cycling define an episode that lasts less than 48 hours before switching to another. So the hypothetical bipolar patient could present in a depressive episode, directly switch to a hypomanic episode, and in less than 48 hours switch to a mixed episode.

It is indeed difficult to define these states and to study them. Moreover, treating ultrarapid cycling bipolar disorder is extremely difficult.

Epidemiology

Bipolar depression (i.e., a depressive episode in either bipolar I or II) typically presents earlier than unipolar depression. Two longitudinal studies—one of 72 children (mean age 12.3 years) diagnosed with major depression followed for 10 years (1) and another of young adults (mean age 23 years) hospitalized with major depression followed for 15 years (2)—showed subsequent rates of hypomania and mania of 48% and 46%, respectively. Men and women are at equal risk for this disorder, and it is found among all races, ethnic groups, and social classes. Bipolar disorder tends to run in families. During the initial assessment of a patient with depression, a positive family history for bipolar disorder strongly suggests that this patient has or will develop a bipolar disorder. The concordance rates for bipolar disorders among monozygotic and dizygotic twins are 33% to 80% and 8% to 23%, respectively. The broad ranges noted occur because the definitions of the disorders have changed over time.

Bipolar Disorders and Suicide

Both attempted and completed suicide are increased in bipolar patients with some estimates of suicide attempts as high as 25% to 50% and the lifetime risk of death by suicide almost 20%. These estimates are often quoted but appear to be overestimates reflecting an inpatient population and not a higher-functioning outpatient population in which suicide rates are much lower. In any case, the rates of completed suicide for people with bipolar disorder at 12% or 20% are significantly greater than in the general population (3). In bipolar patients, suicide is most likely to occur during a depressive or mixed episode. Rapid cycling (i.e., 4 or more mood episodes in a year) bipolar patients are by far the most likely to attempt suicide though not more likely to complete suicide. When noncycling bipolar patients were compared to rapid cycling, the respective suicide attempt rates were 27% and 52%, respectively; when high intent was included, the rates changed to 13% and 30% (nonrapid cycling and rapid cycling) (4). The additional risk factors for suicide reviewed in Chapter 2 also contribute to the baseline risk for bipolar patients.

■ Case-Finding Strategies

In 20% to 25% of depressive episodes, the depression does not represent unipolar depression but is instead a phase of a bipolar disorder. Therefore, when evaluating a patient who is in a depressive episode, the general clinician is required to screen for past episodes of mania or hypomania. This screening can be difficult. Many people suffering with depression do not report past episodes of mania or hypomania either because, being depressed, they lack the cognitive energy to discuss or recall it, or they may simply lack insight into their past manic or hypomanic behavior and fail to recognize it as such. Getting additional history from a family member is very useful, especially if the index of suspicion is high (e.g., positive family history, multiple episodes, irritability). The clinician should consider screening for a history of manic symptoms in the following clinical situations:

- When assessing a depressive episode (see Chapter 3)
- Before initiating an antidepressant (see Chapter 4)
- When excessive irritability or agitation is reported
- When there are multiple episodes of disordered mood
- When there is either a family history of bipolar disorder or any relatives with mood disorders

Discussing current and past episodes of mania or hypomania with patients can be challenging, not because patients resist talking about it, but because patients have trouble describing the symptoms and frequently deny even having them.

For the clinician, avoiding jargon takes some forethought, but fluency comes quickly. One screening strategy for mania focuses on mood lability. The following are examples of good questions:

Do you frequently experience ups and downs in mood?

Do these mood swings seem to occur without cause?

When the screening is positive, the clinician should follow up with more detailed questions using DIGFAST (see Mania and Hypomania earlier in this chapter). Look for false positives, which can commonly occur when screening for mood lability. Know about the "mimics" of bipolar disorders (see Mimics later in this chapter) when screening.

Have there been periods of time when you have felt the opposite of depressed?

Do you have many mood swings for no apparent reason?

Do you need less sleep (or no sleep) and not feel tired?

Do you talk excessively, to the extent of annoying others?

Do you feel like your thoughts are going very fast (racing)?

Do you do anything that could cause problems for you or your family (i.e., reckless driving, spending sprees, sexual behaviors)?

Do other people notice a change in you?

Hirschfeld et al developed a brief survey to detect past episodes of mania in patients presenting in a depressive episode (5). The Mood Disorder Questionnaire (MDQ) consists of 13 yes-no questions that have been validated and used effectively in both mental health specialty and primary care settings. This instrument is useful with either the patient or the patient's family members. When the MDQ screens positive, some experts suggest referring the patient to a psychiatrist to clarify the diagnosis and make recommendations.

Mimics

Mood swings (i.e., lability) and irritability are found in many conditions other than in bipolar disorders. Most of the bipolar "mimics" are related either to substance use or to another psychiatric disorder. However, the clinician should always also consider medical mimics. Delirium from any cause may appear similar to mania, but abnormal or fluctuating levels of consciousness should quickly differentiate it from bipolar disorders. Hyperthyroidism can appear similar to mania during thyroid storm, and CNS lesions or trauma involving the frontal lobes can cause disinhibition and impulsivity. These medical mimics, though significant, occur infrequently when compared to substance-related mimics and other psychiatric disorders.

Substance-Related Bipolar Mimics

Substance abuse frequently co-occurs with bipolar disorders (up to 50% in bipolar II). Substance use itself can induce mood lability, irritability, depression, and impulsive behavior. Determining whether the patient has 1 or 2 disorders (i.e., substance abuse alone vs bipolar disorder plus substance abuse) is only possible if the patient has had a sufficient period of sobriety (at least 3 months) for assessment of symptoms. States of intoxication from substances such as amphetamines or cocaine or withdrawal from substances such as alcohol or benzodiazepines may be indistinguishable from mania. Cannabis withdrawal is seldom recognized, but the person with mood lability who is minimizing his or her daily use as a benign way to "calm down" and be "level" may in fact be managing withdrawal symptoms (e.g., irritability, mood swings). Therapeutic agents including isoniazid, levodopa, and corticosteroids can all induce mania-like states.

Psychiatric Mimics

Borderline personality disorder (BPD) and bipolar disorders (especially bipolar II) both have mood lability as a major component of their diagnoses. Affective instability (i.e., mood lability) occurs in both bipolar disorder and BPD, and both types of patients complain of "mood swings." However, in BPD, the mood swings are typically much more transient, lasting minutes to a day or two, and BPD often includes self-injurious behaviors, like cutting. Distinguishing these two disorders requires a disciplined approach of assessing for *all* the criteria of a mood-disordered episode. If a mood disorder is present, then the clinician should treat it as opposed to ascribing the abnormal symptoms to BPD. Conversely, if the diagnostic criteria for a bipolar disorder are not present, then the clinician should shift his or her treatment focus to BPD. Conversely, if the diagnostic criteria for a bipolar disorder are not present, then shift your treatment focus to BPD. This is an instance in which a psychiatric consultation is definitely indicated because an incorrect diagnosis can have very negative consequences, and treatment of BPD in any case is difficult and complex.

More patients are presenting for treatment of adult attention-deficit/hyperactivity disorder (ADHD). Both bipolar disorders and ADHD share the symptoms of distractibility, impulsivity, and irritability. A history of childhood ADHD is required for the diagnosis of adult ADHD. Of note is a study that found 90% of children who met criteria for bipolar disorder also met the criteria for ADHD (6). However, the opposite was not true—only 25% of children with ADHD also met criteria for a bipolar disorder. The clinician should carefully assess the patient's history and his or her family's history for episodic mood disturbance. (We discuss ADHD and its treatment more fully in Chapter 16.)

Bipolar I, schizophrenia, and schizoaffective disorders have many signs and symptoms that overlap. This is particularly true when bipolar I disorder includes psychosis associated with either its manic or depressive phases or when schizophrenia is accompanied by depressive symptoms or mood lability. Some researchers in the field consider these disorders as parts of the spectrum of a single disorder, while others consider these disorders as separate and distinguishable from each other. Whatever the diagnosis, patients with psychosis have profound dysfunction. Treating them is very difficult, and all patients with bipolar disorders and a history of or current psychosis should be managed by a psychiatrist. (Chapter 11 discusses psychoses including schizophrenia and schizoaffective disorders.)

■ Treatment

Prior to the 1990s, a psychiatrist was typically the primary treating clinician for people with bipolar disorders. This practice pattern existed primarily because managing bipolar patients is complicated, but other factors also facilitated this practice, for example, limited treatment choices (e.g., lithium, carbamazepine, and valproate), the "dangers" of lithium, and greater access to mental health clinicians. The present is very different in 3 respects: (1) the general clinician has assumed a greater (and growing) level of responsibility for the care of bipolar patients; (2) many medications have become available that are perceived as "not dangerous"; and (3) access to mental health services has become more limited. Though many things have changed, the complexity and difficulty of managing patients with bipolar disorders has not.

Currently, there are many treatment options and growing quality data to guide treatment choices. The data have limited clinical applicability, however, because of problems inherent in studying bipolar disorders: patient recruitment is hard, and the recruited patients often differ from those seen in general practice; "gold standards" for the diagnosis do not exist; and studies directly comparing alternative treatments are lacking. Our view is that psychiatrists should still have significant involvement in the management of patients with bipolar disorders. For patients who can be managed as outpatients and do not have acutely evolving symptoms, the psychiatrist's role can be to evaluate the patient in consultation to establish the diagnosis and to recommend treatment. When the patient's symptoms have reached the magnitude of significant functional impairment requiring hospitalization, or when the episode of the bipolar disorder is very complex (e.g., treatment resistant, manic or mixed episodes, psychosis), a psychiatrist should be the primary clinician for treatment. In the following discussion, we assume appropriate access to a psychiatrist and focus our discussion on treatment options for the two most common situations encountered by the general clinician when treating bipolar disorders:

1. Outpatient treatment of bipolar depression (e.g., a depressive episode in bipolar I or II)
2. Maintenance and continuation phase of treatment, in which a psychiatrist is also following the patient

We review the individual medications in more detail in the following section. Discussions involving acute treatment of mania, mixed episodes, and cyclothymia and treatment resistance are beyond the scope of this chapter. We discuss psychotic depression and psychoses in general in Chapter 11.

Treatment Goals

Primary treatment goals include preventing switching and decreasing the frequency of episodes, regardless of their type. The clinician should note that a patient's use of antidepressants complicates treatment because antidepressant use is strongly associated with switching and cycle acceleration. When antidepressants are used, they should be used in the lowest possible doses for the shortest duration. By contrast, the clinician often treats unipolar depression with maximum doses of antidepressants, often chronically.

Treatment of Depressive Episodes in Bipolar Patients

The following treatment options outlined are derived primarily from 3 sets of treatment guidelines from the American Psychiatric Association (APA) (7), the Expert Consensus Series (8), and the Texas Medical Algorithm Project (TMAP) (9). These guidelines take slightly different approaches, so recommendations between the 3 are not in total agreement, but they all share similar guiding principles:

1. Use antidepressants with caution and do not use them alone.
2. Stop the cycling—rely on mood stabilizers.
3. Recommend psychotherapy in maintenance therapy.

Two non-US sets of guidelines from the British Association for Psychopharmacology (BAP) (10) and the Canadian Network for Mood and Anxiety Treatment (CANMAT) (11,12) differ from the US guidelines previously mentioned primarily in their views on antidepressant use. When compared with the US guidelines, both BAP and CANMAT estimate the risk of antidepressant-induced switching as lower and the benefits from antidepressants as higher. However, neither of these guidelines recommend antidepressants as monotherapies in bipolar I depressive episodes. CANMAT, the only guideline to separate bipolar II depression, noted that clinicians *may* recommend monotherapy with an antidepressant if clinicians do so cautiously and with due attention for potential switching states and if they quickly add a mood stabilizer to the medication regimen if switching occurs.

Our view is that the risk of switching a bipolar depressive episode to a mixed, hypomanic, or manic episode with an antidepressant is real and well documented. Even allowing room for debate, the most common treatment for bipolar depression should *not* be an antidepressant used as a monotherapy, but it is. Our advice is this: Do *not* use antidepressants alone to treat bipolar depression.

The FDA currently has approved 9 agents for some aspect of treatment of bipolar disorders, including lithium, anticonvulsants (e.g., divalproex, carbamazepine, lamotrigine), antipsychotics (e.g., olanzapine, risperidone, quetiapine, aripiprazole, ziprasidone), and 1 combination pill (e.g., olanzapine plus fluoxetine). However, FDA indications do not completely describe the therapeutic arsenal since some of the agents are older, long available as generics, and therefore understudied (see Figure 6-1).

Initial Treatment for Bipolar Depression

Lithium is typically given twice a day, started in the outpatient setting at 300 mg at night and titrated up to a blood level of about 0.8 mmol/L (some patients respond to lower doses, and some require doses closer to 1.0 mmol/L). If significant symptom reduction occurs at lower lithium levels, then it is not necessary to titrate up to "therapeutic" serum levels. Serum levels have their greatest utility when assessing nonresponse or toxicity. Lamotrigine is started at 25 mg and titrated up by 25 mg every 2 weeks to a dose between 200 and 300 mg (see Anticonvulsants for more information). Second-line alternatives include combinations of agents in which one agent is always a mood stabilizer. Combinations of lithium plus lamotrigine,

First-Line (Initial) Treatments for Bipolar Depression

Mood Stabilizer* Alone		Antidepressant + Mood Stabilizer		
Lithium	Lamotrigine	Antidepressant + Lithium	Antidepressant +ACD	Antidepressant +Atypical Antipsychotic

Second-Line (Initial) Treatments (Partial or No Response to First-Line Treatment) for Bipolar Depression

Psychiatric consultation and comanagement should be initiated before this line of treatment.)

Mood Stabilizer* Alone	Antidepressant + Mood Stabilizer
- Maximize mood stabilizer - Switch to a different mood stabilizer - Add a second mood stabilizer - Add an antidepressant	- Maximize mood stabilizer - Consider stopping the antidepressant - Switch to different mood stabilizer (use lithium or lamotrigine if not previously used) - Switch to a different antidepressant

ACD = anticonvulsant drug

* Atypical antipsychotics are excluded at this time because the evidence is much stronger for lithium and lamotrigine.

Figure 6-1

lithium plus valproate, lithium plus an antidepressant, and olanzapine plus fluoxetine have all shown efficacy.

If a new depressive episode occurs when the patient is already on a mood stabilizer, then the mood stabilizer is taken up to a maximum dose first; only then should the addition of an antidepressant be considered. "Switching" (from depression to mania) is a risk with all antidepressants, but some carry a greater risk than others. Switches are a little less common in bipolar II (<20%) than bipolar I disorder (30%), so it is reasonable to more readily consider adding an antidepressant when treating bipolar II depression. Tricyclic antidepressants (TCAs) are associated with the highest switch rates (>10%), followed by venlafaxine (10%), monoamine oxidase inhibitors (MAOIs), bupropion (3%), and selective serotonin reuptake inhibitors (SSRIs) (3%). These differences account for the preferential use of bupropion or an SSRI when using an antidepressant in bipolar patients.

Maintenance-Phase and Continuation-Phase Treatment

Prevention and monitoring for early identification of, and intervention for, relapse are important in bipolar disorders because of the high relapse and recurrence rates and frequent noncompliance and because each additional episode is associated with significant morbidity and a poorer prognosis. Relapse and recurrence of mood episodes characterize bipolar disorders. Almost 3 out of 4 patients with bipolar disorders will relapse during maintenance therapy within 5 years of remission or recovery. Preventing relapse and recurrence is the defining goal in maintenance therapy. Monitoring for early relapse is a job shared by the patient, his or her family, and the treating clinician or clinicians. Patients with bipolar disorders frequently have symptoms that do not cross the threshold for a full recurrence. For example, insomnia, irritability, or depressive symptoms may be present for a few days and then subside. These symptoms may be normal, or they may be early markers of relapse and recurrence. Monitoring patients for relapse becomes an exercise in vigilance. Communication among those monitoring for relapse is critical.

   Monitoring for early recurrence of hypomania and mania is often more effectively accomplished by an observer other than the patient (e.g., the patient's family and other clinicians comanaging the patient) (see Box 6-1).

> ### Box 6-1 Monitoring Patients with Bipolar Illness for Early Relapse
>
> **Inquire about and monitor:**
> - Compliance with medication and treatment
> - Side effects of medication
> - Sleep patterns
> - Substance use and abuse
> - Mood changes or lability (e.g., depression, elation, or irritability)
> - Suicidality
> - Recent life events and stresses
> - Blood work (check regularly, depending on medications prescribed, especially if relapse is suspected)
>
> **Educate patient and family about:**
> - Nature of the illness
> - Importance of medication use and compliance
> - Importance of follow-up and continued monitoring
> - Importance of good sleep hygiene (e.g., lack of sleep induces mania)
> - Dangers of substance use (e.g., caffeine, alcohol)
> - Management of work, social activities, and stress

Education about the disorder and the need for medication compliance is an initial focus of treatment and requires consistent reinforcement throughout the course of treatment. All of the clinicians involved with the management of the patient should exchange information regularly. It is important to directly communicate when changes in treatment are made or new symptoms have emerged.

A good communication system allows for *more information* about the patient to emerge. The "system" includes the patient, his or her family or close friends, and other clinicians involved in the management. Enlisting the family early is key. Each extra set of eyes creates opportunities to catch relapse early. For example, substance use may be denied or minimized in one setting and fully revealed in another. Also, a patient may "pull it together" in the clinician's office but be argumentative or irritable at home. The first 6 months of maintenance therapy are the most vulnerable; as routines develop for and around the patient, his or her stability is maximized.

Medications in Maintenance-Phase Treatment

All the guidelines recommend continuing the mood stabilizer, but recommendations regarding antidepressants are mixed. Most experts recommend minimizing the antidepressant's dosage or discontinuing it if possible after depressive symptoms resolve. Lithium is the only drug for bipolar disorder that has been shown to reduce the risk of suicide long term. A meta-analysis comparing 22 studies of long-term lithium maintenance found that, on average, the yearly suicide rate for those on lithium was 0.227% as compared to 1.778% for those not on lithium (13). This represents a significant benefit, but it is by no means a complete prophylaxis, since 0.227% is still more than 13 times the annual suicide rate in the general population (0.017%).

Psychotherapy

Clinicians frequently overlook the psychotherapies in lieu of continually manipulating medications. Though psychotherapies are not indicated as a monotherapy for bipolar disorders, there is mounting evidence of their benefits in maintenance-phase treatments. The psychotherapies studied for bipolar disorders are cognitive behavioral therapy (CBT), interpersonal psychotherapy (IPT), and psychoeducational (PE) modalities. Irrespective of the label, they all share some important common elements:

- Active monitoring for early signs of relapse and recurrence and what to do if it happens
- Strong educational components about bipolar disorders and the need for medications
- Enlisting family and friends into support and monitoring roles
- Promoting behaviors and routines that support remission and recovery and reducing behaviors associated with relapse

In El-Mallakh's and Ghaemi's (2006) book on bipolar depression, they choose to refer to bipolar-specific psychotherapies as BCTs (behavioral cognitive therapy) instead of CBT (14). They put "behaviors" first to emphasize their importance in the treatment of bipolar disorders and to draw a distinction between the emphasis on "abnormal cognitions" in unipolar depression treated with CBT. In both cases the therapies are implemented similarly, but the information and focus is different because the disorders, though similar in some respects, have unique components (e.g., depressed cognitive schemas in unipolar depression and cycling-inducing behaviors in bipolar disorders.)

Colom et al (2003) conducted a particularly well-executed study of over 120 bipolar patients. After remission, half the patients received 21 structured PE group sessions focused on bipolar relapse prevention; the other half received 21 group sessions (with the same psychotherapists) but had no PE about bipolar disorders. At the end of 2 years, the PE treatment groups had between a 40% to 50% relapse rate, and the control groups had an 80% to 85% relapse rate. The differences between the groups started to show around 6 months into the maintenance phase (15). CBTs and IPTs focusing on bipolar relapse and recurrence prevention have shown similar benefits starting to emerge 6 months into the maintenance-phase treatment.

Lifestyle Modifications

Behaviors associated with a regular routine are very important in regulating bipolar symptoms. Think of a "routine" as the opposite of a behavior that promotes cycling. Cycling-inducing behaviors include working erratically, taking medicines irregularly, arguing frequently with family members, and sleeping irregularly. These are associated with relapse and recurrence, whereas routine behaviors facilitate the predictable lifestyle needed to minimize symptoms and detect relapse early.

Regular sleep is particularly important for bipolar patients. Promoting regular sleep-wake schedules is one of the behaviors that clinicians should address early in treatment. Work that requires extra-long or rotating shifts, or traveling through many time zones should be avoided. It frequently takes the clinician's written recommendation to limit travel or modify irregular shifts at work. Activities like staying up late and playing on the computer or watching TV may be difficult to modify but are important to limit. Prospectively monitoring sleep for any changes (once regulated) is a sensitive way to detect early relapse.

Substance use, particularly alcohol, is a frequent issue for people with bipolar disorders. When a patient with unipolar depression (without history of substance misuse) is in remission, an occasional drink is usually not a problem. In bipolar patients, craving a drink or having several drinks is frequently associated with early relapse. It is not clear if alcohol use precipitates bipolar symptoms, or vice versa. Clearly, however, drinking is frequently associated with a relapse of bipolar symptoms. Because the behavior of drinking alcohol is so strongly associated with relapse for many people, we typically advise abstinence from alcohol for bipolar patients.

Pharmacotherapy

The following section describes the pharmacologic options for treating bipolar disorders—including lithium, anticonvulsants, and antipsychotics—in terms of therapeutic effects, side effects, and any special considerations.

Mood Stabilizers

Given the various "controversies" mentioned earlier in this chapter, it should not come as a surprise that there is no agreed-upon definition of a "mood stabilizer." Mood stabilization was initially used to describe lithium because it has beneficial effects on mania and depression and prevents future mood episodes. However, divalproex and carbamazepine are frequently referred to as mood stabilizers but have little or no effect on depression. For the sake of simplicity in this section, we will use the term "mood stabilizer" to describe agents whose primary action includes a short-term or long-term effect of decreasing hypomania and mania. Recall that the discussion of acute mania and its treatment are beyond the scope of this text. (See references for texts that discuss this issue in detail.)

Lithium

Lithium is the oldest mood stabilizer and therefore the one most studied. Its efficacy and side effects are well documented. It is only renally excreted and not hepatically metabolized. Lithium's narrow therapeutic window and toxicity profile make it an agent requiring frequent monitoring, which often occurs in a nonpsychiatric setting. Renal toxicity, hypothyroidism, and diabetes insipidus are some of the most significant adverse reactions. However, benign leukocytosis, tremor, polyuria, polydypsia, and nausea are more commonly seen.

Thiazide diuretics, ACE inhibitors, and high-dose nonsteroidal anti-inflammatory drugs (NSAIDs) should be avoided when using lithium because they increase its blood levels. Before lithium is initiated, the clinician should collect baseline labs for complete blood count (CBC), renal function, and electrolytes. During maintenance treatment, the lithium level, thyroid-stimulating hormone (TSH) level, and renal function should be periodically monitored (at least every 6-12 months when the patient is stable). Electrolytes should also be monitored if the patient is receiving a diuretic, has a medical condition affecting sodium balance, or if lithium-induced polyuria suggests nephrogenic diabetes insipidus. This is often the job of the general clinician. Lithium is typically started at 300 mg at bedtime and titrated up to at least a level over 0.5 mg/dl, with the optimal level in the range of 0.8 to 1.0 mg/dl. Lithium levels over 1.5 mg/dl are toxic. Lithium levels are measured first thing before the morning lithium dose is taken (i.e., at trough levels).

Anticonvulsants

The APA guidelines and the Expert Consensus Series guidelines both recommend the initiation of lithium, carbamazepine (Tegretol), or divalproex (Depakote) before starting an antidepressant in bipolar depression. Carbamazepine was the first anticonvulsant drug introduced for bipolar treatment

> **Box 6-2 Anticonvulsant Mood Stabilizers**
>
> Carbamazepine (Tegretol)
> Divalproex (Depakote)
> Lamotrigine (Lamictal)
> Oxcarbazepine (Trileptal)

in the 1980s. Valproic acid was introduced in 1994. These 2 anticonvulsants have had a significant impact as acute antimanic treatment and prophylaxis against hypomania and mania during the maintenance phase. Virtually every anticonvulsant that now comes to the US market gets tried as a treatment for bipolar disorders. Some have been demonstrated to be effective (e.g., lamotrigine), and some have not (e.g., gabapentin) (see Box 6-2).

Valproic acid, or its most common formulation, divalproex (Depakote), is the most widely used anticonvulsant for bipolar disorders in the United States, with demonstrated efficacy as an antimanic and prophylactic agent. Its major side effects include weight gain, drowsiness, and nausea. Its significant adverse reactions include bone marrow suppression (e.g., anemia, leukopenia, and thromobocytopenia), pancreatitis, and rarely hepatic failure. Baseline labs for CBC and liver enzymes should be collected. Valproic acid causes polycystic ovarian syndrome (PCOS) in some women. The Systematic Treatment Enhancement Program for Bipolar Disorder (STEP-BD) study reported about a 10% occurrence of PCOS in women taking valproic acid (16). Clinicians typically start with 250 mg per day of valproate or a nightly dose of 500 mg of extended release divalproex. The dosage is gradually titrated up until symptoms remit or side effects limit further increases.

Ironically, though carbamazepine was the first anticonvulsant used for bipolar disorder, it was not until 2004 that it was approved by the FDA for the treatment of acute mania. Its potency as prophylaxis during the maintenance phase is similar to lithium. Carbamazepine is started at 200 mg twice daily and titrated up until symptoms abate or it is limited by side effects. The extended-release preparations can be started at night and slowly increased. The "therapeutic" range in serum levels for carbamazepine has been established for seizures, not bipolar disorders. The levels, therefore, only provide a rough guide, with the risk of toxicity increasing at higher levels. The maximum dose should not exceed 1600 mg per day.

The most common side effects of carbamazepine are drowsiness, unsteadiness, headache, and nausea. These are common during initiation of the drug and usually diminish over time. Advancing the dose more slowly can help. Adverse reactions include rare aplastic anemia, hepatic dysfunction, and, more commonly, hyponatremia. Carbamazepine induces its own metabolism by cytochrome enzymes, thereby reducing its blood levels. These should be checked 2 to 4 weeks after a steady state is achieved. Carbamazepine can induce the metabolism of other drugs, too. Notably, oral contraceptives can have their effectiveness reduced because of lower blood levels. This is particularly important because carbamazepine is associated with significant birth defects. Prior to initiating carbamazepine, the clinician should collect baseline labs for CBC, liver enzymes, and electrolytes.

Oxcarbazepine (Trileptal) is a metabolite of carbamazepine, and they are structurally very similar. However, liver toxicity has not been reported with oxcarbazepine as it has with carbamazepine. Oxcarbazepine is not FDA approved for bipolar disorders but has clinically been used as a carbamazepine substitute. The evidence for its effectiveness is limited, though the APA included it in its guidelines. It is typically initiated at 150 mg twice daily and titrated up. The maximum dose is 1800 mg per day.

Side effects of oxcarbazepine include dizziness, double vision, nausea, and vomiting. Like carbamazepine, these tend to be transient but may persist at higher doses. Oxcarbazepine is not associated with many serious adverse events but can cause significant hyponatremia in a minority of patients. No pretreatment labs are currently recommended.

Recent evidence supports the use of lamotrigine (Lamictal) as a monotherapy for depression in patients with bipolar I and II, and it is FDA approved for the maintenance treatment of bipolar disorders. It appears to have the greatest antidepressant effect of the currently available anticonvulsants. It does not cause significant weight gain or nausea. It does, however, cause the potentially life-threatening skin reaction, Stevens Johnson Syndrome-Toxic Epidermal Necrolysis (SJS-TEN) in a minority of cases. Lamotrigine seems to cause a benign rash in up to 10% but causes SJS-TEN in 0.01% of cases. Raising the dosage very slowly reduces the incidence of the rash. A typical starting dose is 25 mg once daily for 2 weeks, increased to 50 mg for 2 weeks, and so forth. Most patients will respond to doses between 100 and 200 mg, but higher doses of 300 to 400 mg are not uncommon.

Though gabapentin (Neurontin) was initially used as an antimanic agent, controlled studies have not demonstrated it to be effective. Some clinicians believe it has a role as a second anticonvulsant for bipolar patients with significant anxiety. Topiramate (Topamax), like gabapentin, was hoped to have antimanic properties, but the trials to date have not supported this. Topiramate has some appeal as an add-on to conventional mood stabilizers in treatment-resistant bipolar disorder because it is the only anticonvulsant that tends to cause weight loss rather than weight gain.

Great caution should be used when prescribing mood stabilizers to women of childbearing years because of known and potential risks to the fetus. Valproic acid and carbamazepine are associated with spina bifida, and lithium is associated with Ebstein anomaly. Carbamazepine can reduce levels of oral contraceptives, making them ineffective. Women of childbearing years who are pregnant or wish to become pregnant need a detailed psychiatric and obstetric consultation to weigh the risks and benefits in this very complicated, high-risk situation. This is discussed in detail in Chapter 16, which includes women's mental health issues.

Atypical Antipsychotics
Clozapine was the first "atypical" antipsychotic. It is very effective in treatment-resistant bipolar disorder. Its many side effects and adverse reactions have

> **Box 6-3 Atypical Antipsychotics**
>
> Aripiprazole (Abilify)
> Clozapine (Clozaril)
> Olanzapine (Zyprexa)
> Risperidone (Risperdal)
> Quetiapine (Seroquel)
> Ziprasidone (Geodon)

limited its use. However, the use of newer atypical antipsychotics is increasing for the treatment of bipolar disorders, in particular for bipolar depressions and maintenance-phase treatments (see Box 6-3). All of the atypical antipsychotics reviewed here have FDA-approved indications as antimanic and maintenance agents. Olanzapine-fluoxetine (Symbyax) and quetiapine (Seroquel) have received FDA approval for the treatment of bipolar depression, as well. The older typical antipsychotics have been used this way for many years as well. (Antipsychotics and their side effects are discussed in detail in Chapter 11.)

Antidepressants
The use of antidepressants should be approached cautiously when treating bipolar depressions. As previously noted, most guidelines recommend the combination of a mood stabilizer and an antidepressant with the mood stabilizer initiated first. Most experts would recommend the initiation of an SSRI or bupropion as first-line antidepressant augmentation. For a more detailed discussion of individual antidepressant agents, see Chapters 4 and 5.

KEY POINTS

- Bipolar disorders are essentially mood disorders characterized by episodes of depression and episodes of either mania or hypomania.
- The first presentation of manic or hypomanic symptoms is likely to be recognized in the primary care setting.
- Mania is severe and lasts at least 7 days, whereas hypomania lasts 4 days and some normal functioning occurs.
- Screening for mania and hypomania should occur whenever the diagnosis of major depression is noted, especially if an antidepressant is initiated.
- A depressive episode may switch to a manic or hypomanic episode if an antidepressant is used alone, without a concurrent mood stabilizer.
- Lithium, valproic acid, and carbamazepine are the mood stabilizers that make up the first-line treatment for mania.

- There is growing evidence to support lamotrigine as a first-line treatment for bipolar depression.
- Newer agents including mood stabilizers and atypical antipsychotics have a growing role in the treatment of bipolar disorders.

REFERENCES

1. Geller B, Zimerman B, Williams M, et al. Bipolar disorder at prospective follow-up of adults who had prepubertal major depressive disorder. *Am J Psychiatry.* 2001;158:125-127.

2. Goldberg JF, Harrow M, Whiteside JE. Risk for bipolar illness in patients initially hospitalized for unipolar depression. *Am J Psychiatry.* 2001;158:1265-1270.

3. Dutta R, Boydell J, Kennedy N, et al. Suicide and other causes of mortality in bipolar disorder: a longitudinal study. *Psychol Med.* 2007;37:839-847.

4. Coryell W, Solomon D, Turvey C, et al. The long-term course of rapid-cycling bipolar disorder. *Arch Gen Psychiatry.* 2003;60:914-920.

5. Hirschfeld RM, Cass AR, Holt DC, et al. Screening for bipolar disorder in patients treated for depression in a family medicine clinic. *J Am Board Fam Pract.* 2005;18:233-239.

6. Carlson GA. Mania and ADHD: comorbidity or confusion. *J Affect Disord.* 1998; 51:177-187.

7. American Psychiatric Association. Practice guideline for the treatment of patients with bipolar disorder (revision). *Am J Psychiatry.* 2002;159:4.

8. Keck PE Jr, Perlis RH, Otto MW, et al. The expert consensus guideline series: treatment of bipolar disorder. *Postgrad Med Special Report.* 2004;1-120.

9. Suppes T, Dennehy EB, Swann AC. Report of the Texas Consensus Conference Panel of Medication Treatment of Bipolar Disorder 2000. *J Clin Psychiatry.* 2002; 63:288-299.

10. Nutt DJ. British Association for Psychopharmacology Consensus on the treatment of bipolar disorder. *J Psychopharmacol.* 2003;17(2):147.

11. Canadian Network for Mood and Anxiety Treatments (CANMAT) guidelines for the management of patients with bipolar disorder: consensus and controversies. *Bipolar Disord.* 2005;7(suppl 3):5-69.

12. Canadian Network for Mood and Anxiety Treatments (CANMAT) guidelines for the management of patients with bipolar disorder: update 2007. *Bipolar Disord.* 2006;8:721-739.

13. Tondo L, Hennen J, Baldessarini RJ. Lower suicide risk with long-term lithium treatment in major affective illness: a meta-analysis. *Acta Psychiatr Scand.* 2001; 104(3):163-172.

14. El-Mallakh RS, Ghaemi SN. *Bipolar Depression, A Comprehensive Guide.* Arlington, VA: APPI Press; 2006.

15. Colom F, Vieta E, Martinez-Aran A, et al. A randomized trial on the efficacy of group psychoeducation in the prophylaxis of recurrences in bipolar patients whose disease is in remission. *Arch Gen Psychiatry.* 2003;60(4):402-407.

16. Joffe H, Cohen L, Suppes T, et al. Valproate is associated with new-onset oligoamenorrhea with hyperandrogenism in women with bipolar disorder. *Biol Psychiat.* 2006;59(11):1078-1086.

KEY REFERENCES

Akiskal HS, Bourgeois ML, Angst J, et al. Re-evaluating the prevalence of and diagnostic composition within the broad clinical spectrum of bipolar disorders. *J Affect Disorder.* 2000;59:S5-S30.

Bowden CL. Strategies to reduce misdiagnosis of bipolar depression. *Psychiatr Serv.* 2001;52:51-55.

Das AK, Olfson M, Gameroff MJ, et al. Screening for bipolar disorder in a primary care practice. *JAMA.* 2005;293:956-963.

Ghaemi SN, Boiman EE, Goodwin FK. Diagnosing bipolar disorder and the effect of antidepressants: a naturalistic study. *J Clin Psychiatry.* 2000;61:804-808.

Gijsman HJ, Geddes JR, Rendell JM, et al. Antidepressants for bipolar depression: a systematic review of randomized, controlled trials. *Am J Psychiatry.* 2004;161: 1537-1547.

Goldberg JF, Harrow M, Whiteside JE. Risk for bipolar illness in patients initially hospitalized for unipolar depression. *Am J Psychiatry.* 2001;158:1265-1270.

Hirschfeld RM, Bowden CL, Gitlin MJ, et al. Practice guideline for the treatment of patients with bipolar disorder (revised). *Am J Psychiatry.* 2002;159:1-50.

Leverich GS, Altshuler LL, Frye MA, et al. Risk of switch in mood polarity to hypomania or mania in patients with bipolar depression during acute and continuation trials of venlafaxine, sertraline, and bupropion as adjuncts to mood stabilizers. *Am J Psychiatry.* 2006;163:232-239.

Perlis RH, Brown E, Baker RW, et al. Clinical features of bipolar depression versus major depressive disorder in large multicenter trials. *Am J Psychiatry.* 2006; 163:225-231.

Phelps JR, Ghaemi SN. Improving the diagnosis of bipolar disorder: predictive value of screening tests. *J Affect Disord.* 2006;92:141-148.

Rush AJ. Introduction. Bipolar disorder: origin, recognition, and treatment. *J Clin Psychiatry.* 2003;64:4-8.

Suppes T, Leverich G, Keck P, et al. The Stanley Foundation Bipolar Treatment Outcome Network, 2: demographics and illness characteristics or the first 261 patients. *J Affect Disorder.* 2001;67:45-59.

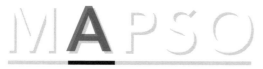

Anxiety
Disorders

A

Panic Disorder and Generalized Anxiety Disorder

■ Panic and Generalized Anxiety Disorders and the General Clinician

A

Physical symptoms can occur in all psychiatric disorders but are particularly significant in generalized anxiety disorder (GAD) (e.g., muscle tension, fatigue, insomnia) and panic disorder (e.g., chest pain, dyspnea, choking, hot flushes) because they are actually part of the diagnostic criteria for these disorders. Their somatic nature helps explain why so many people with these disorders visit their general clinicians. A diagnostic difficulty for both the patient and general clinician is that the presenting problem is often not "anxiety" per se. Introducing the idea of an anxiety disorder as the cause of physical symptoms is not typically intuitive for the general clinician or for the patient. Patients can feel dismissed if their physical symptoms are ascribed to a psychiatric disorder. The general clinician should be well versed in detecting when somatic symptoms may be manifestations of a psychiatric disorder; this is especially common in the focus of this chapter, GAD and panic disorders, where worry and fear are also present with physical symptoms.

Anxiety, Angst, and Fear

There is some confusion and misperception surrounding anxiety disorders, in part because the word *anxiety* is nonspecific and has different meanings depending on the context. Anxiety, like depression, can represent a normal state, an abnormal symptom, a set of clinical syndromes, or the full criteria for a DSM-IV disorder. In addition, though patients may deny "anxiety," they may admit to nervousness, insomnia, worry, stress, muscle tension, nausea, sweating, or spells of overwhelming fear.

Freud originally used the word *angst*, which was later translated to *anxiety*. Freud viewed angst as a state related to fear, where fear refers to the set of feelings and sensations we have when exposed to a real and present danger outside of us, and angst or anxiety refers to the same set of feelings and sensations induced by a nameless, imagined, wholly internal danger. So someone experiencing angst or anxiety will have the same autonomic responses as someone confronting a bear face-to-face, but the "bear" is inside the individual, ill defined, and usually nameless. For the patient, the experience of angst or anxiety-related symptoms is "real," but the cause is imagined or ill defined. The general clinician and patient's challenge is sorting through these real experiences and symptoms that do not typically have an external cause.

Panic Disorder

Essential Concepts and Terms

Panic disorder involves recurrent, unexpected panic attacks and a persistent concern about having another panic attack. A *panic attack* is a classic example of Freud's concept of angst. All the *fight-or-flight* signals spontaneously erupt, but there is nothing to fight or flee from. Panic attacks, like other anxiety symptoms, may occur in isolation, represent a medical or substance-induced condition, be a manifestation of another psychiatric disorder, or be part of an anxiety disorder (e.g., panic disorder). Though panic attacks occur abruptly, they are typically short-lived, reaching a peak within 10 minutes. According to the DSM-IV, a patient must have at least 4 of the signs and symptoms in Box 7-1.

> **Box 7-1 Panic Attack: Signs and Symptoms**
>
> A panic attack includes 4 or more of the following symptoms that occur together and peak at 10 minutes:
>
> - Palpitations
> - Sweating
> - Trembling
> - Shortness of breath
> - Choking
> - Chest pain
> - Nausea or sudden gastrointestinal symptoms
> - Dizziness or lightheadedness
> - De-realization
> - Fear of losing control
> - Fear of dying
> - Paresthesia
> - Chills
> - Flushing

In a classic story, after learning from his clinician that his severe chest pain and shortness of breath were due to a myocardial infarction, a patient replies, "I am so relieved, I thought my panic attacks had returned." With panic disorder, distress and dysfunction occur not only because of the discomfort associated with panic attacks but also because patients often avoid situations where a panic attack may occur, both in hope of preventing an attack and because of their embarrassment over panicking in public . This concern over the occurrence of the next panic attack often leads to more distress and dysfunction than the actual panic attack. Initially, people avoid specific situations where escape is difficult (e.g., a bridge or elevator), but the avoidance can progress and generalize. The result is people staying in the confines of their homes and avoiding going out. The term agoraphobia is used when avoidance has generalized to this extreme.

Agoraphobia, fear of the *agora*, or open places, accompanies panic disorder 33% to 50% of the time. Patients with agoraphobia have marked anxiety about being in a place or situation in which escaping or obtaining help may be difficult if a panic attack were to occur. In essence, agoraphobia is a phobic avoidance of panic attacks; that is, the patient's anxiety intensifies to such a degree with the thought of or exposure to a possible panic attack that all possible measures are taken to avoid this exposure. Agoraphobia can exist without panic, but, clinically, agoraphobia almost always follows panic disorder. Panic disorder with agoraphobia is associated with more morbidity and treatment resistance than panic disorder alone. Even after the panic symptoms abate, agoraphobia often persists. Pharmacological treatments are effective for panic attacks but are not usually effective for agoraphobia. The longer panic disorder is left untreated, the higher the likelihood of agoraphobia developing, which underlines the importance of early diagnosis and treatment of panic disorder. Agoraphobia should be distinguished from other phobias (e.g., specific phobias or social phobia, discussed in Chapter 9); social isolation in major depression, paranoid disorders, or avoidant or schizoid personality disorders; and avoidant behavior in post-traumatic stress disorder (PTSD).

Epidemiology

Panic attacks are fairly common, with a lifetime prevalence of at least 10% to 30%, but only 1% to 3% of the general population will actually develop panic disorder. Within the primary care setting, the prevalence of panic disorder ranges as high as 8% to 11%. The high reported prevalence of panic disorder in the primary care setting is partially attributable to the fact that >90% of patients with panic disorder present with somatic complaints.

Most panic attacks occur in younger people. There is a bimodal distribution for the age of onset, one peak in late adolescence and another in the mid-30s. The 1-month prevalence of panic disorder in the general population has been reported to be 1% to 2% for men and 2% to 5% for women. Women are twice as likely to have not only panic but also panic with agoraphobia.

People with panic disorder utilize health care services much more often than the general population; one reason for this is that many patients with panic disorder initially present to the emergency department (ED) with somatic symptoms, most often chest pain. In a 1996 study, 25% of patients with chest pain who presented to the ED had panic disorder, although in 98% of the patients with panic disorder, the panic disorder was not recognized by the ED cardiologist (1).

Palpitations in the absence of a cardiac arrhythmia are common in patients with panic disorder. Studies with ambulatory monitoring of both cardiac and normal patients show that the correlation between the perception of palpitations and actual cardiac rhythm irregularities is weak (2). Patients who have had panic attacks become sensitized and hypervigilant for irregularities in bodily functioning and therefore tend to overperceive and overinterpret normal and minor abnormal somatic sensations.

Comorbidities

Panic attacks can occur in people with no disorder, with any of the other major anxiety disorders, or with major depression. Panic disorder, however, is most often comorbid with either GAD or major depression. When associated with PTSD, obssessive-compulsive disorder (OCD), or phobias, panic attacks are often triggered by specific events. For example, panic attacks may occur in a patient with PTSD when exposed to a reminder of the traumatic experience; in a patient with OCD with a contamination obsession who is forced to use a dirty public bathroom; or in a patient with social phobia who is faced with having to give an important public presentation. In these instances the patients have panic attacks but not panic disorder. Management is focused on the primary disorder (e.g., PTSD, OCD, social phobia), and the panic attack is only a symptom.

The rate of overlap between GAD and panic disorder is 40%, and this overlap is even higher between GAD and panic attacks. In the past, GAD and panic disorder were considered the same disorder because the symptoms overlap to such a high degree. GAD, however, occurs in a pure state in a significant minority of cases. An important distinction is that, in panic disorder, the patient worries primarily about having a recurrent panic attack, whereas in GAD worry is generalized and may cover many aspects of the person's life.

Panic attacks and panic disorder frequently co-occur with major depression; about 50% of patients with panic disorder have major depression, and 30% to 40% of patients with major depression have recurrent panic attacks. Recognizing the co-occurrence of a mood disorder with panic disorder should influence treatment choice. When a mood disorder occurs with panic disorder, resolution of all symptoms may take longer and require more than one agent.

Case-Finding Strategies

Screening for Panic Disorder

Patients can misinterpret attempts to screen for panic attacks as attempts to *discount* their "physical" symptoms as "all in their heads." Referring to the possible panic attack as an "episode" or "spell" helps shift the focus from the pursuit of the cause of the symptoms to the process of the description of the symptoms.

For example, a 24-year-old woman is having recurrent spells of intense nausea, sweating, shortness of breath, and faintness. The initial medical evaluation is negative, and you have a high index of suspicion that these symptoms represent a panic attack. She wants to know what is wrong with her. Your reply should include something like, "It's not clear what has caused these spells, but let's back up and review all of the things that happen during one of them."

Screening questions would include the following:

Can you describe the entire spell from start to finish?

Was it triggered by something?

How long did it last?

What did you do?

How did it make you feel?

A

Were there any other symptoms or feelings you had?

When was the first time you had an episode like this?

Where you scared by this?

What were you afraid would happen?

The more associated physical symptoms the patient reports that are consistent with panic attacks and the more preoccupied the patient is with fear of having another "spell," the more likely panic disorder is the correct diagnosis.

Mimics

The lifetime prevalence of a panic attack is between 10% and 30%, but the vast majority will not have any underlying psychiatric disorder. The first task is to carefully assess for either a medical condition or substance that could have caused the symptoms (e.g., secondary panic attacks), but frequently no cause can be found (see Box 7-2).

Substance-induced panic attacks are associated with either acute effects (e.g., intoxication) of stimulating substances (e.g., sympathomimetics including beta-2 agonists, caffeine, nicotine, amphetamines, cocaine) or the withdrawal of sedating substances (e.g., benzodiazepines, alcohol). The sudden cessation of an antidepressant or the acute effects of a decongestant taken in combination with coffee may also induce panic-like symptoms.

Box 7-2 Medical Mimics of Panic Attacks

- Cardiac disorders (e.g., supraventricular tachycardia [SVT], angina)
- Pulmonary disorders (e.g., asthma attacks, chronic obstructive pulmonary disease [COPD], pulmonary embolism)
- Endocrinopathies (e.g., hyperthyroidism, pheochromocytoma, carcinoid)
- Neurological disorders (e.g., akathisia, tremors, brain tumor)
- Abuse of substances (e.g., cocaine, amphetamines, ecstasy, alcohol withdrawal)
- Caffeine (overconsumption)
- Medications (e.g., antidepressants, theophylline, sympathomimetics)
- Herbal supplements (e.g., herba mate, ma huang)
- Electrolyte abnormalities (e.g., hypocalcemia, hypomagnesemia)
- Sleep disorders (e.g., sleep apnea, night terrors)

Most "guilty" substances are discovered by carefully reviewing with the patient *all* substances recently ingested (or stopped) in the last 24 to 48 hours. If the index of suspicion remains high, then collecting a urine drug screen and collateral information is often helpful.

Some serious medical conditions may be mistaken for panic attacks. Any person experiencing a sudden onset of extreme symptoms and fear may, in fact, be having a myocardial infarction, vertigo, near syncope, cardiac arrhythmia (i.e., supraventricular tachycardia), hypoglycemia, asthma, or a pulmonary embolus.

■ Generalized Anxiety Disorder

Essential Concepts and Terms

People with GAD have excessive anxiety (i.e., worry) that generalizes to most areas of a person's life, including the smaller, mundane areas (e.g., tardiness, the weather, everyday encounters). People with GAD recognize that their worrying is excessive and have trouble controlling it. GAD is the combination of this excessive worrying plus other symptoms (see the list that follows) resulting in significant functional impairment. GAD is a chronic disorder with periodic exacerbations; symptoms tend to worsen during times of stress and lessen when the stressful period has passed. Despite the high prevalence and significant morbidity in GAD, detection rates remain low. Further, when GAD is detected, treatment is often inadequate.

According to the DSM-IV, symptoms of GAD must meet the following guidelines:

- It must be present for more days than not and for a 6-month period.
- It must not be caused by a medical condition or substance.
- The worrying is associated with at least 3 of the following symptoms:
  - Restlessness or feeling "keyed-up" or "on edge"
  - Easy fatigability
  - Difficulty concentrating or the mind going blank
  - Irritability
  - Muscle tension
  - Sleep disturbance
- The worry is not limited to key features of another disorder such as worrying about the next panic attack (i.e., panic disorder), worrying about social encounters and embarrassment (i.e., social phobia), worrying about contamination (i.e., OCD), or worrying about gaining weight (i.e., eating disorders).

Epidemiology

The lifetime prevalence for GAD in the general adult population ranges from 4% to 7%. Within the primary care setting, 8% of patients meet criteria for GAD, making it the most common anxiety disorder in primary care. One urban primary care clinic reported a rate over 14%. In one longitudinal study, only 15% had a full remission of 2 months or longer in the first 2 years of the study, and at 5 years only 38% had had a full remission (3). Women have approximately twice the lifetime prevalence rate (6.6%), and as many as 10% of women over age 40 have GAD. Though the average age of onset for GAD is 21 years, unlike the other anxiety disorders, symptoms of GAD may first develop and progress later in life, too. High prevalence rates continue into the fifth decade of life (4). It is not clear why this prevalence pattern occurs, but it is in part due to the chronic and relapsing nature of GAD.

A

Comorbidities

GAD is also frequently found to co-occur with another psychiatric illnesses. The lifetime comorbidity rate for all psychiatric disorders and GAD is 90%. Depression co-occurs with both GAD and panic disorder more than 50% of the time. Also, anxiety is a common symptom in major depression though not listed as a criterion in the DSM-IV.

Case Study

Mr A is a 36-year-old man who presents with worsening fatigue, poor sleep, and poor concentration. There are increased stressors at home, including financial and marital pressures. His son was recently diagnosed and treated for attention-deficit/hyperactivity disorder (ADHD). Mr A is hopeful that this will help decrease stress at home. He adds, "My son is a lot like me. Could I have ADHD too?" However, in elementary school Mr A was an "excellent student with perfect behavior," unlike his son. Mr A further notes: "I know I'm the nervous type, but I'm afraid something is really wrong." Mr A's history, exam, and labs reveal that his diastolic blood pressure is elevated to 96 mm Hg, and he is 125% of his ideal body weight. Basic labs including thyroid, electrolytes, CBC, cholesterol panel, and liver profile only show elevated cholesterol.

Case-Finding Strategies

The predominance of somatic symptoms in GAD can confound diagnosis. People with GAD usually present with physical symptoms, not "anxiety." Because GAD is such a mixed bag of worry, physical symptoms, impairment, and comorbid disorders, it is little wonder that it is so hard to recognize, diagnose, and treat. Recognition and diagnosis are improved by the general clinician's considering the possibility of GAD in the following patient presentations:

- Multiple unexplained physical symptoms (e.g., insomnia, fatigue, headache)
- Irritability
- A self-described "nervous type"
- Concerns about adult attention deficit disorder (ADD)
- Features of both depression and anxiety

Making a definite diagnosis is difficult when there are numerous factors that could be causing or contributing to Mr A's symptoms. As with all psychiatric symptoms, the first step is to consider medical conditions and substances that may cause or contribute to his symptoms (see Box 7-2). The possibility of ADHD is very small given a normal childhood history (see Chapter 16 for more information about adult ADD). That leaves unexplained somatic symptoms (i.e., fatigue, poor sleep, and poor concentration) in a 36-year-old man who is self-described as nervous and has trouble relaxing.

Two screening instruments for GAD (the GAD-7 and its ultra-brief cousin, the GAD-2) have been recently developed. The GAD-7 has good sensitivity and specificity for GAD. However, the first 2 questions of the GAD-7 (i.e., the GAD-2) served equally well for screening not only for GAD but also for 3 other anxiety disorders (i.e., panic disorder, PTSD, and social

---

Table 7-1 GAD-7*

Over the last 2 weeks how often have you been bothered by the following problems?

	Not at all (Score 0)	Several days (Score 1)	More than days (Score 2)	Nearly every day (Score 3)
Feeling nervous, anxious, or "on edge"	☐	☐	☐	☐
Not being able to stop or control worrying	☐	☐	☐	☐
Worrying too much about different things	☐	☐	☐	☐
Having trouble relaxing	☐	☐	☐	☐
Being so restless that it is hard to sit still	☐	☐	☐	☐
Becoming easily annoyed or irritable	☐	☐	☐	☐
Feeling afraid as if something awful may happen	☐	☐	☐	☐
Total score	☐	☐	☐	☐

*Note that the first 2 items are the GAD-2.

phobia). Scores for the GAD-7 and GAD-2 range from 0 to 21 and 0 to 6, respectively. Cut-off scores of greater than or equal to 7 and 2, respectively, had sensitivities >90% for any anxiety disorder. Higher scores were associated with greater specificities for the 4 anxiety disorders noted but especially for GAD (see Table 7-1) (5).

Further questioning should be directed toward GAD or GAD plus another comorbid illness, particularly depression. When considering the diagnosis of GAD, clinicians should ask additional case-finding questions about worrying, including the following:

A

Are you a worrier?

Do others think you worry a lot?

How often do you find yourself thinking about your worries?

Can you control your worrying, or is it hard to turn off?

Next, explore for other symptoms like restlessness, muscle tension, and irritability, as well as comorbid disorders like mood disorders (e.g., major depression dysthymia, bipolar II), other anxiety disorders (e.g., panic disorder, PTSD, OCD, and phobias), and substance abuse.

■ Treatment of Panic Disorder and Generalized Anxiety Disorder

Both psychotherapy and pharmacotherapy are effective treatments for panic disorder and GAD. The best-studied psychotherapy for both GAD and panic disorder is cognitive behavioral therapy (CBT). The pharmacotherapy choices include benzodiazepines, antidepressants (selective serotonin reuptake inhibitors [SSRIs] and tricyclic antidepressants [TCAs]), buspirone, and newer agents. Given that the general clinician will mostly see situations in which there are comorbid disorders and treatments that are needed long term, patients should have individualized management that is collaboratively pursued with the treating mental health clinician. The treatment suggestions described here are offered as guides and not rigid rules because most of the evidence underlying this guidance is based on studies of patients with "pure" disorders that are treated short term.

Psychotherapy

CBT is the psychotherapy most effectively used to treat both GAD and panic disorder. The evidence is clear that CBT is effacacious in treating GAD and panic disorder (6). CBT is used alone and in combination with pharmacologic agents. However, consistent evidence is lacking demonstrating the superiority of one approach (i.e., CBT vs pharmacotherapy vs combined treatment), which may partly be due to the high comorbidity that occurs in these 2 disorders (7).

An understanding of CBT is important not only so that the general clinician can explain how it can help the patient but also because the general clinician can use its basic principles to guide his or her interactions with the patient. The following discussion of CBT focuses on its application to panic disorder, but the descriptions can be easily adapted for GAD. CBT was also discussed in Chapter 4 as an initial treatment for unipolar depression.

Cognitive Behavioral Therapy

CBT is a symptom-oriented approach as opposed to an insight-oriented approach. The American Psychiatric Association's (APA) *Practice Guideline for the Treatment of Patients with Panic Disorder* presents 5 key components in CBT for panic disorder that are beneficial elements in any treatment of panic disorder, even if the patient is not in formal CBT with a psychotherapist (see Box 7-3).

> **Box 7-3 Key Concepts in CBT for Panic Disorder**
>
> ---
>
> 1. Education
> 2. Continuous panic monitoring
> 3. Breathing retraining
> 4. Cognitive restructuring
> 5. Exposure to fear cues

Education of the patient about his or her illness, treatment options, and expectations are starting points in the management of any disease. The educational approach for panic disorder should highlight the interaction between the physical or biological nature of panic and the associated thoughts, feelings, and behaviors. Breaking the symptoms down into these components and looking for any triggers begins the process of the patient gaining control over the panic attacks. This approach helps patients understand and conceptualize their symptoms and dysfunction as a treatable disorder instead of feeling out of control or discounted because the symptoms are "all in my head."

Continuous panic monitoring is basically a symptom diary. The purpose is for the patient to gather information about the nature and circumstances of the attacks, including length, duration, and frequency of panic attacks; cues or possible triggers; and the thoughts and feelings experienced before and during the attacks. These thoughts or cognitions are often distorted, and when patients confront this distortion, they can better understand and subsequently control their symptoms.

Breathing retraining is based on the rationale that hypocapnia and respiratory irregularities are underlying factors in the development of panic. By practicing measured, controlled breathing at the onset of a panic attack, patients may be able to prevent full attacks. It is most helpful for patients who hyperventilate during or prior to panic attacks.

Cognitive restructuring encompasses techniques used to identify and counter fear associated with bodily sensations. It is characteristic in panic disorder for the patient to think catastrophically, meaning that he or she overestimates the probability of a negative consequence (e.g., a heart attack). After the feared catastrophic situation is identified, the patient is invited to gather reality-based information to test and counter the distorted catastrophic estimation.

Exposure to fear cues is the final and central component of CBT. After the patient has done the work previously noted, it is important to confront the panic attacks and associated triggers. This has to be done carefully because if it is done prematurely and panic persists, it further reinforces the association of the fear cues and panic. Such a process of CBT takes time and skill.

Some patients wrongly believe that a referral to a therapist for CBT will mean lying on a couch talking about their mothers, a media caricature of psychotherapy. The general clinician can allay this concern by emphasizing that CBT is a highly specific educational process that is symptom-oriented and behavior-oriented and focuses on current relief, not on looking for an explanation in the distant past.

A

Pharmacotherapy

Benzodiazepines

Benzodiazepines have been effectively used to treat anxiety symptoms and anxiety disorders since the 1960s, and a large body of evidence has amassed supporting their safety and efficacy. Thus, benzodiazepines are the most frequently prescribed medication for GAD and panic disorder. The Harvard/Brown Anxiety Research Project (HARP), an ongoing prospective naturalistic study of patients with anxiety disorders, found that alprazolam was the most frequently used drug by patients with GAD (31%), followed by clonazepam (23%) (8). The same study, which also followed patients with panic disorder, reported that benzodiazepines were the most commonly used class of medications in panic disorder despite the introduction of SSRIs during the time period of the study. These observations are consistent with our clinical observations that, for many patients with anxiety disorders, benzodiazepines are effective and safe for long-term use.

The long history of benzodiazepines includes negative experiences resulting from erroneous prescription as monotherapy for depression by general clinicians and from patient misuse, abuse, and overdose. Regrettably, the negative experiences have led some patients and clinicians to totally avoid this class of medications. On the other hand, benzodiazepines are not completely benign, and their cavalier prescription can be harmful.

Which Patients Should Be Prescribed Benzodiazepines?

This question is easier to approach when restated as, Who should *not* get benzodiazepines? Central to this question is the abuse and addiction potential of benzodiazepines. Some patients (and clinicians) avoid benzodiazepines because they "don't want to get addicted to them." Addiction refers to the misuse of an agent for pleasure or escape and is not synonymous with tolerance and withdrawal. Withdrawal symptoms may occur in anybody who takes a sufficient dose of a benzodiazepine daily for an extended period of time and stops abruptly. Benzodiazepines do not typically cause addiction or misuse in patients who are not vulnerable to addiction (i.e., those without past and current substance abuse). In our experience, most patients without a substance abuse history who receive daily long-term treatment with benzodiazepines tend to develop a tolerance to sedation side effects but not the therapeutic effects, and thus their dose remains stable over time. The APA's Task Force on Benzodiazepine Dependence, Toxicity, and Abuse states: "There are no data to suggest that long-term therapeutic use of benzodiazepines by patients commonly leads to dose escalation or to recreational abuse" (9). However, caution is warranted because of the high rates of comorbid substance abuse in patients with GAD or panic disorder; in the case of alcohol abuse, the co-occurrence rates are 10% to 20% for those with GAD and 37% for those with panic disorder. Nevertheless, the majority of patients with anxiety disorders do not have comorbid substance abuse and may be appropriate candidates for benzodiazepines. Careful screening and collateral history will identify most cases of substance abuse, but if in doubt, wait and reassess. You do not lose the option to prescribe a benzodiazepine later. It has been our clinical experience that, ironically, many patients who would benefit most from taking benzodiazepines are often so anxious about the potential for addiction that they refuse them or underutilize them when prescribed.

Selecting a Specific Benzodiazepine and Dosing

Benzodiazepines provide antianxiety effects essentially from the first dose. This rapid onset of action makes them particularly valuable early in treatment when patients are typically most symptomatic. A benzodiazepine is not required during initiation of an antidepressant, but it is helpful for those patients requiring immediate symptom relief (e.g., many panic disorder patients). In appropriate patients, benzodiazepines are often initially co-administered with an antidepressant for several weeks or months and then tapered off when the therapeutic effects of the antidepressant have occurred. This approach is used in both GAD and panic disorder (see Table 7-2).

Intermediate half-life benzodiazepines (most often clonazepam) are preferred to short half-life agents (e.g., alprazolam, lorazepam) when daily dosing is to occur. The short half-life agents do not stay in the patient's system long enough and therefore require dosing several times per day. When this happens for an extended period of time, patients can experience withdrawal symptoms between doses and think that their anxiety symptoms have recurred. This can lead to dose escalation driven by withdrawal symptoms that are mistaken for core symptoms of the disorder. As a general rule, short half-life drugs pose a higher addiction risk than longer half-life drugs in the same family. Therefore, we recommend intermediate half-life agents like clonazepam. Its longer half-life and few active metabolites make it ideal. It is started at either 0.5 mg at night or twice daily and is titrated up slowly until symptoms remit. Sedation is the dose-limiting side effect.

Table 7-2 Benzodiazepines in the Treatment of Anxiety Disorders

Frequently Used Agents	Half-life*	Active Metabolite(s)	Onset of Action†	Comments
Alprazolam (Xanax)	6-12 hours	1	Rapid	
Lorazepam (Ativan)	>6 hours	Few but significant	Rapid	Primary active metabolite half-life is 50 hours
Clonazepam (Klonopin)	18-24 hours	None	Delayed	
Alprazolam XR (Xanax XR)	11-16 hours	1	Delayed	
Diazepam (Valium)	>24 hours	Many	Rapid	Primary active metabolite half-life is 100 hours
Chlordiazep-oxide (Librium)	>24 hours	Many	Delayed	

*Includes active metabolites.
†Onset of action is a balance between lipid solubility and time-to-peak level.

A

A short half-life agent like alprazolam is very effective for use as needed. Its rapid onset of action can abort escalating panic anxiety symptoms. Like our patient who has carried it in her purse for 10 years, the knowledge that a fast-acting agent is available has been very reassuring and therapeutic in her case, even when not actually taken. The ability to "medically" abort an attack empowers patients to go places they may otherwise avoid. Alprazolam may be used for this purpose because it has a rapid onset of action. When "as needed" use of a short half-life benzodiazepine turns into multiple doses daily, it is time to consider switching to a longer-acting intermediate agent or adding an antidepressant.

Some patients do extremely well on just a benzodiazepine. Most do not increase the dose unless acute stressors exacerbate their anxiety symptoms. An intermediate half-life benzodiazepine is appropriate in these situations. A trial of antidepressants may allow the benzodiazepine dose to be reduced or eliminated, but the HARP study of long-term use of benzodiazepines in patients with panic disorder demonstrated that some patients stop the antidepressant but continue the benzodiazepine and do very well.

Discontinuing a Benzodiazepine

Discontinuing a benzodiazepine is challenging, especially when either GAD or panic disorder is present. Benzodiazepines have an almost immediate anxiolytic effect, as opposed to over a few weeks for antidepressants, and rapidly condition the patient to expect the effect. Complicating things further, physiological dependence (without abuse) often occurs and withdrawal presents in a significant proportion of patients when they discontinue use too abruptly.

The length of the taper and the use of accompanying medications depend on several variables:

- The duration of benzodiazepine treatment
- The daily dose
- The half-life (including active metabolites)
- The patient's willingness to stop the benzodiazepine

Some advocate for a relatively quick taper if the patient has been on the benzodiazepine for 6 months or less. In our experience, dependence sometimes occurs quickly, and even short courses (2-4 weeks) of benzodiazepines can occasionally require tapers that are ultimately longer than the treatment. Exacerbation of symptoms is most likely during 3 time periods: the day of the dose reduction, the last half of the taper, and the first week after the taper is completed. Often an antidepressant (e.g., a TCA, an SSRI, or a newer agent) is added to the patient's drug regimen before tapering the benzodiazepine. This allows the new agent to get into the patient's system and have a maximum effect before the benzodiazepine is removed. Sometimes difficulty with discontinuation of a benzodiazepine signals a possible undetected comorbid condition (e.g., substance abuse, another anxiety disorder). As mentioned earlier, referral to a psychiatrist can be helpful to determine if long-term continuation of the benzodiazepine may be indicated or if a comorbid condition has been missed.

Antidepressants

The word "antidepressant" is a misnomer, especially when used to describe their use to treat anxiety disorders. In any case, antidepressants as a group have become the backbone of psychopharmacology for the treatment of GAD and panic disorder, whether in pure or comorbid states. The categories of antidepressants include SSRIs, TCAs, and other agents. Multiple studies have shown that SSRIs and TCAs effectively treat GAD and panic disorder.

Antidepressant side-effect profiles do differ among the agents, and there are individual patient variations in vulnerability to side effects even within a class (see Chapter 4 for a complete discussion of antidepressants and their side-effect profiles). One complication in the use of antidepressants to treat anxiety disorders is that antidepressants can induce or transiently increase anxiety symptoms (e.g., panic symptoms), especially when the dose is increased too quickly or started at too high a dose. The initial activation or stimulation sometimes seen with antidepressant initiation, with both SSRIs and TCAs, can feel like an exacerbation of anxiety symptoms. Typically, a "start low and go slow" approach is warranted in the treatment of anxiety disorders. An early negative effect can lead to abortive discontinuation of medication before a therapeutic effect can develop. Especially in the highly anxious, somatically sensitive patient, start at the lowest antidepressant dose possible and alert the patient about the side effects. Simple reassurance is usually enough to help the patient through the first 7 to 10 days. If the patient has had past treatment failures or has symptoms so acutely distressing that an SSRI alone is likely to fail, then starting a benzodiazepine first or in conjunction with the antidepressant is a good strategy.

A

SSRIs
More easily tolerated than TCAs and without the sedation or risks for withdrawal and addiction of benzodiazepines, SSRIs have become the drugs of choice in GAD and panic disorder. Though not all SSRIs carry GAD and panic disorder as indications in the *Physicians' Desk Reference* (PDR), experts consider all SSRIs as first-line treatments for these disorders. As in depression, there are claims of differential efficacy or onset of action for the various SSRIs. Most of these claims are put forth by the pharmaceutical industry. Clinical experience and evidence from numerous studies, however, suggest equal efficacy and onset of action among the SSRIs.

Tricyclic Antidepressants
Before SSRIs, TCAs were the drugs of choice for panic disorder and GAD. Imipramine has the largest body of evidence supporting its use. TCAs, like SSRIs, are considered effective as a class in the treatment of panic disorder and GAD. We use nortriptyline primarily because it has a more favorable side-effect profile than amitriptyline and imipramine.

Venlafaxine and Duloxetine
Venlafaxine and duloxetine are serotonin-norepinephrine reuptake inhibitors (SNRIs). Their serotonin-increasing effects are similar to SSRIs, but they have an additional norepinephrine-increasing effect. Venlafaxine is FDA approved for both GAD and panic disorder, and duloxetine is FDA approved for GAD. We use both in the treatment of GAD and panic disorder, particularly in patients who fail to respond to an SSRI.

Newer Antidepressants
Mirtazapine has some antianxiety properties, and there is evidence supporting its efficacy in both GAD and panic disorder, but it is not FDA approved for treatment of GAD or panic disorder. Given so many other choices, we consider it a second-line or third-line option. Bupropion is the one antidepressant that does not appear beneficial in treating primary anxiety disorders, perhaps in part because it is the most stimulating of the antidepressants.

Monoamine Oxidase Inhibitors

Monoamine oxidase inhibitors (MAOIs) have been effectively used in the treatment of refractory panic disorder and other anxiety disorders (e.g., social phobia). They require medication and dietary restrictions, which have limited their current use to patients who are refractory to other medications.

Buspirone

Buspirone (BuSpar) is in a distinct class of agents called azapirones. Azapirones are structurally and pharmacologically unrelated to benzodiazepines but still have antianxiety properties that effectively treat GAD. The effect, however, is delayed by up to 2 weeks, which limits its usage for some patients wanting immediate or as-needed benefits. Buspirone's lack of immediate effect, tolerance, or withdrawal means it carries no addiction potential, making it a good choice in the patient who has a significant history for substance abuse or where a benzodiazepine is contraindicated. Though effective for GAD in clinical studies, buspirone has not been found to be effective in panic disorder.

Treatment of Subsyndromal Anxiety

Psychotherapy is always an option whether the patient has a syndromal or subsyndromal condition (see Box 7-4). Patients who are experiencing anxiety in response to specific stressors and have the willingness and capacity to participate make excellent candidates for psychotherapy. There are numerous effective psychotherapies, including cognitive behavioral psychotherapy, interpersonal psychotherapy, and supportive psychotherapy. All are effective in relieving symptoms, especially when associated

> **Box 7-4 General Principles for the Treatment of Subsyndromal Anxiety**
>
> ---
>
> - Find out if the current symptoms are residual symptoms of a full criteria disorder.
> - Ask if there is a family history of anxiety disorders.
> - Use a conservative approach.
> - Provide close follow up.

with specific stressors. Other nonpharmacological treatments, especially relaxation techniques, can be particularly helpful for the anxious patient. Guided imagery, meditation, and breathing exercises are all examples of relaxation techniques that can be employed when the patient experiences these symptoms and in their prevention.

Pharmacologic treatment for isolated anxiety symptoms primarily consists of antihistamines and benzodiazepines. Hydroxyzine and diphenhydramine both have anxiolytic effects, which are often associated with sedation and anticholinergic side effects (e.g., dry mouth, sedation, urinary retention). Antihistamines are good short-term medications when used at night in younger patients who can tolerate their side effects, but they are not a good choice in older patients because their anticholinergic properties can cause delirium, constipation, and urinary retention. Short half-life benzodiazepines, as previously described, are ideal for isolated anxiety symptoms (e.g., anxiety over a presentation or fear of air travel). If the patient genuinely requires daily benzodiazepines, this indicates that a full syndromal anxiety disorder is probably present and may indicate the need for long-term treatment.

■ Treatment of GAD Comorbid with Depression

A

Antidepressants are beneficial in the treatment of all of the anxiety disorders and unipolar depressive disorders. When an anxiety disorder and depression are comorbid, SSRIs are most commonly used, but evidence is lacking to support any particular monotherapy (e.g., SSRIs, SNRIs, TCAs) or combination over another. The general management strategy utilizes the same approaches as outlined previously:

- Start at a low dose and go slowly.
- Consider the co-administration of an intermediate-acting benzodiazepine (e.g., clonazepam) and an antidepressant.
- Consider a sedating antidepressant (e.g., a TCA or mirtazapine) alone or in combination. This may be helpful.

KEY POINTS

- Anxiety disorders are common; about 1 in 4 Americans will meet criteria for diagnoses of anxiety in their lifetime.
- Anxiety disorders are much more likely to co-occur with another disorder (especially depression) than to occur alone or in a "pure" state.
- There are numerous conditions that mimic panic attacks.
- Panic attacks can occur in all the anxiety disorders and major depression, not just panic disorder.
- Cognitive behavioral therapy (CBT) is the psychotherapy with the most evidence supporting its effectiveness in panic disorder and GAD.
- Benzodiazepines have an important role in the management of GAD and panic disorder.
- Antidepressants are the first-line treatments for GAD and panic disorder.

REFERENCES

1. Fleet RP, Dupuis G, Marchand A, et al. Panic disorder in emergency department chest pain patients: prevalence, comorbidity, suicidal ideation, and physician recognition. *Am J Med.* 1996;101:371-380.

2. Barsky AJ. Palpitations, arrhythmias, and awareness of cardiac activity. *Annals Int Med.* 2001;134:832-837.

3. Yonkers KA, Dyck IR, Warshaw M, et al. Factors predicting the clinical course of generalised anxiety disorder. *Brit J Psychiat.* 2000;176:544-549.

4. Kessler RC, Wittchen HU. Patterns and correlates of generalized anxiety disorder in community samples. *J Clin Psychiatry.* 2002;63(suppl 8):11-16

5. Kroenke K, Spitzer RL, Williams JBW, et al. Anxiety disorders in primary care: prevalence, impairment, comorbidity, and detection. *Ann Int Med.* 2007;146:317.

6. Hunot V, Churchill R, Silva de Lima M, et al. Psychological therapies for generalised anxiety disorder. Cochrane Database Syst Rev. 2007 Jan 24;(1):CD001848.

7. American Psychiatric Association. Practice guidelines for the treatment of patients with acute stress disorder and posttraumatic stress disorder. *Am J Psychiatry.* 2004;161:3-31.

8. Salzman C, Goldenberg I, Bruce SE, et al. Pharmacologic treatment of anxiety disorders in 1989 versus 1996: results from the Harvard/Brown anxiety disorders research program. *J Clin Psychiatry.* 2001;62(3):149-152.

9. *Benzodiazepine Dependence, Toxicity, and Abuse: A Task Force Report of the American Psychiatric Association.* Washington, DC: American Psychiatric Association; 1990.

Key References

Bass C, Mayou R. ABC of psychological medicine-chest pain. *BMJ.* 2002;325(7364): 588-591.

Dammen T, Bringager CB, Arnesen H, et al. A 1-year follow-up study of chest-pain patients with and without panic disorder. *Gen Hosp Psychiatry.* 2006;28(6):516-524.

Dyck IR, Phillips KA, Warshaw MG, et al. Patterns of personality pathology in patient with generalized anxiety disorder, panic disorder with and without agoraphobia and social phobia. *J Pesonal Disord.* 2001;15:6071.

Fricchione G. Generalized anxiety disorder. *N Engl J Med.* 2004;351:675-682.

Goldenberg IM, White K, Yonkers K, et al. The infrequency of "pure culture" diagnoses among the anxiety disorders. *J Clin Psychiatry.* 1996;57(11):528-533.

Katon WJ. Panic disorder. *N Eng J Med.* 2006;354:2360-2367.

Keller MB. Social anxiety disorder clinical course and outcome: review of Harvard/Brown Anxiety Research Project (HARP) findings. *J Clin Psychiatry.* 2006;67:14-19.

Kessler RC, Berglund P, Demler O, et al. Lifetime prevalence and age-of-onset distributions of DSM-IV disorders in the National Comorbidity Survey Replication. *Arch Gen Psychiatry.* 2005;62:593-602.

Olfson M, Shea S, Feder A, et al. Prevalence of anxiety, depression, and substance use disorders in an urban general medicine practice. *Arch Fam Med.* 2000;9:876-883.

Wang PS, Lane M, Olfson M, et al. Twelve-month use of mental health services in the United States results from the National Comorbidity Survey Replication. *Arch Gen Psychiatry.* 2005;62:629-640.

Wittchen HU, Hoyer J. Generalized anxiety disorder: nature and course. *J Clin Psychiatry.* 2001;62:15-19.

Post-traumatic Stress Disorder

▮ Post-traumatic Stress Disorder and the General Clinician

A

Most cases of post-traumatic stress disorder (PTSD) are encountered in civilians. The major problem in diagnosing PTSD is that it often does not "look" or "act" like PTSD when we see it clinically. People seldom come in complaining of PTSD, and when they do, it usually is *not* PTSD. Typically, a person comes in with physical complaints or manifestations of a comorbid disorder (e.g., major depression, substance abuse). PTSD is comorbid with another disorder 80% of the time. The high prevalence of physical symptoms further contributes to its underrecognition and partially explains the higher prevalence rates of PTSD in primary care settings when compared to the general population.

PTSD, like syphilis 75 years ago, is only recognized when the seemingly disparate symptoms are considered as possibly coming from a single underlying cause and then diagnosed when the etiology is actively identified. In both cases, once the general clinician recognizes that the symptoms are all associated with a common etiology, he or she can readily make the diagnosis by searching for evidence of spirochetes in syphilis or the traumatic stressor and its sequelae in PTSD.

For the general clinician, the "essentials" of PTSD include understanding the terms, concepts, and diagnostic criteria for PTSD; knowing the situations that require a high index of suspicion for PTSD; learning screening questions and strategies to find PTSD when it is present; and knowing some basic concepts in the treatment of PTSD. Though the treatment of PTSD is considered complicated, it is the knowledge and skills required to recognize and diagnose PTSD that require the general clinician's greatest effort and attention.

▮ Essential Concepts and Terms

The Traumatic Event—Stressor Criterion A

The concept of a traumatic stressor is central to understanding PTSD, which is the only psychiatric disorder to have such importance placed on the etiological event. The DSM-IV has 2 stressor criteria (criterion A) that the traumatic event must fulfill: the person must be directly exposed to a catastrophic event involving an actual or perceived threat to life or limb of himself or herself or others *and* during the event, the person must experience extreme fear, helplessness, or horror.

"Conditional risk" is used to convey the dose-response relationship between the traumatic stressor and the likelihood of causing PTSD. For example, the conditional risk for a traumatic stressor (e.g., rape) is the percentage derived from the number of people exposed to the particular trauma who get PTSD divided by the total number of people exposed to this kind of trauma.

$$\text{Conditional risk for trauma A} = \frac{\text{Number exposed to trauma A who get PTSD}}{\text{Total number exposed to trauma A}}$$

The conditional risks of developing PTSD for adolescent survivors of motor vehicle accidents, adult female victims of rape, and prisoners of war have been reported as 20%, 38%-49%, and 67%, respectively. Specific characteristics of the trauma determine the magnitude of the "dose" and the likelihood of subsequent PTSD:

- The duration, frequency, and intensity of the trauma (e.g., ongoing physical abuse of a battered spouse)
- The unpredictability or uncontrollable nature of the trauma (e.g., a natural disaster like a hurricane or tornado)
- Bodily injury (e.g., assault, motor vehicle accident, surgery)
- Victimization either sexually or by violence (e.g., torture)
- Tragic, sudden loss of a loved one (especially a child or spouse)

Despite having experienced significant traumas, most people do not develop PTSD. For example, a sample of Oklahoma City bombing survivors was followed for subsequent psychiatric disorders. Though all experienced significant distress, many did not experience a psychiatric disorder that met the full criteria. In fact, 70% of those who survived the bombing (and who did not have a premorbid psychiatric disorder) did not develop any psychiatric disorder, including PTSD.

There are risk factors that increase a person's vulnerability to PTSD following a traumatic event. The major risk factors that increase the likelihood of subsequent PTSD are listed in Box 8-1.

Box 8-1 PTSD Risk Factors

- Great severity of the stressor*
- Poor social support*
- Subsequent life stressors*
- History of prior traumatic event*
- Past history of childhood abuse
- Female
- Comorbid psychiatric disease
- Family history for psychiatric disease

*These factors carry the highest risk.

Symptom Sequelae of PTSD

If a traumatic event meets the stressor criterion A, then the diagnosis of PTSD requires that the patient also have symptoms from 3 criteria categories:

- Re-experiences (criterion B)
- Avoidance-numbing (criterion C)
- Increased arousal (criterion D)

These categories include symptoms found in the other anxiety disorders: the worry and irritability of generalized anxiety disorders (GAD), the intensity and panic of panic disorder (PD), the obsessions (about the trauma) like in obsessive compulsive disorder (OCD), and the phobic avoidance (of triggers) seen in phobias. It is no wonder that the "forest" is hard to see (see Box 8-2).

> **Box 8-2 Key Symptoms of PTSD**
>
> *PTSD is characterized by persistent symptoms falling into 3 groups:*
>
> - **Re-experiences**: intrusive thoughts, nightmares, flashbacks
> - **Avoidance**: isolation, numbness, avoidance of thoughts and triggers
> - **Hyperarousal**: jitteriness, hyper-vigilance, insomnia, irritability

Re-experiences—Criterion B

The unwelcome re-experiences of the traumatic event are perhaps the most distinctive and readily identified symptoms associated with PTSD. The word "flashback" has entered modern vocabulary, and most patients understand what it means. The re-experiences can range from recollections that are hard to keep out of one's mind, to events where the person literally re-experiences all the sensations and associated fear of the trauma, including visual and auditory memories of the trauma. PTSD memories feel different than memories from nontraumatic events; they feel as though they just happened or are still happening. A patient described it once by saying, "It's like it got stuck on the screen of my computer. I cannot get it into the 'memory.'" Re-experiences can be so vivid that the patient may experience them as hallucinations. This, combined with the tendency in PTSD to dissociate, may lead to a mistaken diagnosis of a primary psychotic disorder. Associations and reminders connected to the traumatic event can trigger the re-experiences. Some of the triggers are obvious, like an anniversary or a certain location, but some triggers are subtler, like smells or noises. Patients with PTSD often take extreme measures to avoid the triggers, and they profoundly reshape their lives.

Avoidance and Numbing—Criterion C

These symptoms include all of the cognitive and behavioral strategies used by trauma survivors to diminish the likelihood that they will come in contact with or feel the effects of stimuli (i.e., triggers) associated with the traumatic event. Cognitive avoidance strategies range from making conscious efforts not to think about the traumatic event to less conscious strategies such as shutting down emotionally and avoiding all feelings (i.e., numbness).

Many people with PTSD do not associate their current symptoms with the traumatic event. In fact, when directly asked, many trauma survivors report horrific traumas with little or no affect. Sometimes their affect can appear inappropriate, especially if the patient giggles or trivializes the traumatic experience. Avoidance symptoms contribute to the underrecognition of PTSD because trauma survivors either avoid any connections with the trauma or "normalize" their responses when asked about it. It is not uncommon for patients who eventually get treatment to report that the reason for not getting treatment sooner was that they did not think they had a "problem" stemming from the traumatic event or that they were responding "normally" to the event.

Hyperarousal—Criterion D

These symptoms are what make PTSD an anxiety disorder that overlaps with other anxiety disorders, particularly GAD and PD. Insomnia, irritability, muscle tension, and poor concentration are all examples of the hyperaroused state in PTSD. Trauma survivors have described themselves as "always on the ready." A patient who had chronic insomnia but slept well during the day eventually revealed that her experience was that repeated sexual assaults always occurred at night when people were asleep. She felt she "was only safe when the sun was up." Her sedating nighttime medications were discontinued, and she eventually changed to working a night shift and sleeping during the day.

Additional Criteria

Time—Criterion E

The diagnosis for PTSD requires that the symptoms persist for at least 1 month after the traumatic event; symptoms meeting criteria A through D but lasting less than a month are called acute stress disorder (ASD). This is an arbitrary cutoff of doubtful clinical relevance when a patient clearly has all of the symptoms previously outlined and significant functional impairment (i.e., criterion F).

Functional Impairment—Criterion F

All psychiatric disorders require significant functional impairment as part of their criteria. The functional impairment from PTSD, however, may not be obvious when first considered. As previously noted, one of the central features of PTSD is avoiding triggers (i.e., criterion C) associated with the event, so the patients with PTSD often resist the efforts of a clinician to directly associate their symptoms of insomnia, nausea, and poor concentration with the traumatic event. Similarly, patients with depression may also resist the idea that their fatigue, insomnia, and pain are symptoms of the depression but eventually realize the connection as symptoms abate with treatment. While some patients resist the diagnosis of any psychiatric disorder, the avoidant cognition and behavior in PTSD constitute additional barriers to its diagnosis.

Physical Symptoms Associated with PTSD

The somatic complaints associated with patients with PTSD are of particular significance to the general clinician. Patients with PTSD are more likely than other patients to have *amplification* of physical symptoms or *unexplained* physical symptoms (e.g., somatization). Though somatic symptoms are part of other psychiatric disorders (e.g., weight loss and sleep disturbance in major depression; muscle tension and decreased concentration in GAD), somatic symptoms are at least 2 times as likely to be associated with PTSD than with another psychiatric disorder. The most common somatic symptoms found in a study of Gulf War veterans with PTSD were fatigue, sleep disturbance, joint pain, memory loss, headache, and difficulty concentrating. Though the reason or reasons for the connection between traumatic events and somatic symptoms is speculative, some posit a connection between an impaired ability to differentiate relevant from irrelevant stimuli and a tendency to focus on and misinterpret somatic sensations (1).

Clinical Course

The clinical course of PTSD is varied. Some trauma survivors try to maintain their functioning through emotional numbing. This is initially protective but eventually can lead to a delayed onset of PTSD symptoms. However, when PTSD follows ASD, the greatest symptom severity occurs in the immediate aftermath of the trauma. In the latter, more "classic" clinical course of PTSD, symptoms typically decrease within the first year, and most individuals who spontaneously recover usually do so within 3 months. About 30% to 50% of patients with PTSD will recover in 1 year. In any traumatized symptomatic population, patients who develop PTSD will eventually recover 75%-80% time (2). However, 20%-25% of patients with PTSD will develop a chronic relapsing and remitting course. One study of WWII prisoners of war showed that 50% of survivors still had PTSD symptoms 40 years later (3).

The classic clinical course, however, is not the one typically seen by the general clinician. The clinical course of undetected PTSD in primary care is one that can easily span years. PTSD patients frequently have many somatic complaints and have developed comorbid disorders like major depression. The traumatic event may have occurred before the patient entered the general clinician's practice, and the clinician may be unaware that the traumatic event occurred. In this scenario, the patient does not reference the traumatic event, as previously noted. For these reasons, we recommend actively screening all patients for significant past traumas when performing an initial evaluation or yearly physical (see sections on screening strategies later in this chapter).

Epidemiology

Initially, PTSD was only recognized in combat soldiers. Now it is recognized as primarily a civilian disorder with 90% of the cases of PTSD found in the general population. Between 50% and 90% of the general population are exposed to a trauma sufficient to cause PTSD. Fortunately, while many people are exposed to severe traumas, the vast majority do not develop PTSD.

PTSD has lifetime prevalence rates between 1% and 4% in the general population. However, prevalence rates in the primary care setting typically range between 9% and 12%, and a recent Robert Wood Johnson survey of a public hospital clinic found 19% of men and 27% of women met criteria for PTSD (4). Yet the vast majority of these patients' PTSD symptoms remain unrecognized and untreated.

PTSD and Suicide

Suicidal ideation is particularly frequent in PTSD, more prevalent than in any of the other anxiety disorders. Persons who have PTSD are 6 times more likely than the general population to attempt suicide. The risk factors associated with suicide (see Chapter 2) are additive and should be evaluated and directly addressed in the patient's management.

Comorbidity

Comorbidity with other psychiatric disorders is the rule rather than the exception. A comorbid condition exists in more than 80% of PTSD cases. Major depression and substance abuse are the most frequent comorbid psychiatric conditions. Recognizing the common overlapping symptoms of PTSD and its comorbid disorders is helpful for the general clinician because it prospectively creates associations with clusters of symptoms that may represent PTSD (see Table 8-1).

■ Case-Finding Strategies

The general clinician should focus his or her attention on 2 screening strategies. The first screening strategy is employed with a new patient with whom the general clinician has no prior relationship from which to draw. In this situation, the focus is on screening for a traumatic event that could have produced or did produce PTSD in the past. Knowing that such an event occurred gives the general clinician a "heads up" for the possibility of PTSD and the increased vulnerability the patient has if exposed to

Table 8-1 The Great Masquerader: PTSD

Symptom of PTSD	Mimic
Avoidance	Depression, Social phobia, Agoraphobia
Panic attacks	Panic disorder
Irritability	Personality disorder, GAD, Bipolar disorders
Psychotic-like states	Schizophrenia, Mania, Psychotic depression
Excessive worry	GAD
Phobic avoidance	Social phobia
Obsessions	OCD

A

another significant trauma. The second strategy is a disorder-defining approach, in which the general clinician suspects PTSD and is actively pursuing the diagnosis. The general clinician requires skills in exploring for the 3 major symptom categories of PTSD (i.e., re-experiences, avoidance, hyperarousal).

Screening for Traumatic Events

Discussing traumas with patients requires a degree of sensitivity and practice as well as an understanding of PTSD. The general clinician is searching for an event that was extreme and overwhelming. Also, the patient may be trying to avoid (consciously and unconsciously) memories or feelings about the event. We have found that a clear and direct approach works best.

> *Have you ever had a very traumatic experience like a car accident, an assault, or the sudden death of someone close to you?*

If the patient becomes upset or tearful, then a validating statement is helpful:

> *I can see this is painful for you to talk about. Let's focus on how you have coped with it.*

If a patient expresses appropriate sadness about a tragic event, this is a good sign that they have integrated some of the emotion associated with the experience. On the other hand, a patient who describes a horrific event (e.g., rape, assault, a near-fatal accident) with no expression of feeling may be demonstrating the avoidance and emotional numbing associated with PTSD. Occasionally, people who have experienced a traumatic event may almost automatically launch into a very detailed description of the event. Though these details are very important, opening them up and addressing them in an initial screening is not recommended. Much like the previous validating statement, the general clinician can redirect the patient with a statement like this:

All of the details of this event are extremely important, but today let's focus on the bigger picture of how you are doing so we can make an appropriate plan.

When a general clinician discovers that a significant traumatic event has occurred, he or she should remember that PTSD is still relatively unlikely, especially if the patient is minimally symptomatic or asymptomatic. A brief sentence of education explaining PTSD is helpful as a segue to the next set of questions:

Some people who experience traumatic events, as you have, develop a disorder called post-traumatic stress disorder. I am going to ask some specific questions to see if this has occurred.

Screening for Re-experiences

Screening for re-experiences follows the same approach used in screening for trauma. Be clear and direct:

Do you have bothersome memories, dreams, or images of the event? How have you tried to lessen these?

Screening for Avoidance Symptoms

A hallmark of PTSD, and the source of much functional impairment, is the patient's modification of his or her life to avoid thoughts or feelings associated with the trauma. Understanding the magnitude of the measures taken to avoid the triggers is a good indication of the level of impairment.

Do you try to block out thoughts or feelings related to the trauma?

Do you avoid places or situations that remind you of the trauma?

Do you have any blank spots in your memory of the trauma?

However, much of the screening for avoidance symptoms is accomplished by observation, not inquiry. The numbing and lack of expressed emotions are typical manifestations of avoidance symptoms. Questions that explore how much contact is made with other people and what activities are engaged in are very helpful. For example, after a motor vehicle accident, a person with PTSD may avoid the area of the accident, and in more extreme instances, the patient may generalize the symptom to all travel and stay in the house.

If patients have had re-experiences of the trauma, assess their responses. Often, intense physiological responses occur, like a fight-or-flight response. Trauma survivors usually know the triggers that will precipitate re-experiences and will avoid them.

Screening for Hyperarousal

Like screening for symptoms of avoidance, symptoms of increased arousal are found more often with observation than inquiry. Increased states of arousal may be present if the patient seems restless, has trouble sitting still, or startles easily. Insomnia, trouble concentrating, and irritability can also indicate an increased state of arousal. If symptoms are not obvious on observation, then explore what happens when the patient is confronted with a trigger. A report of panic-like symptoms is consistent with hyper-arousal and PTSD.

A

■ Treatment

Treatment for PTSD cannot be characterized by a single approach or method. Given the complex, heterogeneous nature of PTSD, a collaboration is required between the general clinician and a psychiatrist and/or a psychotherapist. The primary care clinician should first educate the patient about PTSD as a disorder and its relationship with symptoms and impairment. Next, the clinician should clarify the target symptoms and review how treatment should affect the patient. No single treatment works in all cases. However, successful treatments typically include 2 or more clinicians working collaboratively with the patient. The general clinician's role includes facilitating the treatment with a psychiatrist and a psychotherapist or comanaging with a psychotherapist, in which the general clinician provides medication management. A low threshold for referral to a psychiatrist early in the treatment is advised to establish the diagnosis and recommend the most appropriate treatment, including careful attention to psychiatric comorbidity. The following section reviews basic medications and psychotherapy used in the management of PTSD.

Psychotherapy

Psychotherapy plays a significant role in the treatment of PTSD. Patients may not be receptive to psychotherapy at certain stages of treatment, but most benefit at some time during the course, and bringing it up early clearly communicates its value even if it is not utilized initially. Many different forms are available, and no single psychotherapeutic approach has proven better than another in PTSD. In our opinion, the choice of the individual psychotherapist is more important than the type of psychotherapy. An experienced psychotherapist who has worked with trauma survivors is the best choice. A novice who offers poorly executed psychotherapy or a psychotherapist who is overly aggressive therapeutically can harm the patient by exacerbating symptoms and in some cases, recapitulating the traumatic event in some real or symbolic way. Skilled psychotherapists recognize the dangers and benefits of psychotherapy in PTSD and tune their technique to the individual patient. Identifying good psychotherapists prospectively requires some investment of time, but the dividend is effective treatment for your patients with PTSD.

Pharmacotherapy

Patients with sustained symptoms of PTSD can benefit from the use of medications. Often several trials of different medications and combinations of medications are required to achieve sufficient response. In the last decade, selective serotonin reuptake inhibitors (SSRIs) have become the backbone of pharmacotherapy in PTSD. However, most other antidepressants (tricyclic antidepressants [TCAs], monoamine oxidase inhibitors [MAOIs], serotonin-norepinephrine reuptake inhibitors [SNRIs; e.g., venlafaxine and duloxetine], newer antidepressants [e.g., mirtazapine]), as well as antipsychotics and antiepileptic agents have all been used with success in treating PTSD.

SSRIs and TCAs

As with the other anxiety disorders, an antidepressant (usually an SSRI or SNRI) should be started at the lowest dose and titrated up slow to avoid side effects and exacerbation of the hyperarousal symptoms. If the therapy is successful, medication should be continued for at least 1 year. Older antidepressants (e.g., TCAs, MAOIs) have also been effective in the treatment of PTSD, especially when severe comorbid depression is present or the initial antidepressant has failed. For discussions of the individual antidepressants, including dosing and adverse reactions, see Chapter 4.

Other Antidepressants

Trazodone is frequently used in PTSD to help with insomnia and unpleasant nightmares (a common form of re-experience). It is typically used in combination with another agent (e.g., SSRI, SNRI). Many patients cannot tolerate the sedation accompanying higher doses of trazodone (e.g., >150 mg); however, some patients with PTSD not only tolerate higher doses but also have very positive responses. In our experience, doses of 300 to 400 mg are not uncommon. (Adverse reactions and other general information regarding trazodone are found in Chapter 4.)

Mirtazapine (Remeron) is a newer antidepressant that is FDA approved for the treatment of depression but has been found to help patients with comorbid anxiety disorders. Small studies support its use in PTSD, and clinical experience is growing with this agent. Given its sedating effects, it is typically given at night and titrated up. (Adverse reactions and other general information regarding mirtazapine are found in Chapter 4.)

Antiepileptic Drugs

Antiepileptic drugs (AEDs) have been successfully used in the treatment of PTSD. The typical target symptom for these agents is irritability, which can manifest as explosive symptoms. These agents are only used in augmentation and are not monotherapies for PTSD. (For information regarding the individual AEDs, including dosing and adverse reactions, see Chapter 6.)

Antipsychotics

The use of *antipsychotics* is increasing in patients with PTSD. They seem to be particularly effective in suppressing intrusive thoughts and nightmares. Like anticonvulsants, antipsychotics are an add-on therapy and not a monotherapy. Their common sedating effect makes them a good choice to use at night. Frequently, these medications can be tapered off or reduced after remission is achieved, and another agent, usually an antidepressant, is continued into maintenance-phase treatment. (For information regarding the individual antipsychotics, including dosing and adverse reactions, see Chapters 6 and 11.)

A

Less-Effective Medications

Bupropion (Wellbutrin) is not effective for "pure" PTSD, although it is an effective treatment for major depression. Some clinicians have seen PTSD symptoms exacerbated (e.g., re-experiences and increased arousal) with bupropion and reserve it for augmentation of another antidepressant in patients with major depressive disorders (MDD) and PTSD. When used to augment treatment for depression, it is titrated up slowly with a single morning dose, typically starting with 100 mg of the sustained-release preparation. (For general information regarding bupropion, including dosing and adverse reactions, see Chapters 4 and 5.)

Though *benzodiazepines* are effective in the other anxiety disorders, placebo-controlled trials suggest that they should be used sparingly in PTSD because they are either ineffective or make the symptoms worse, perhaps by disinhibiting re-experiencing symptoms. However, they are effective for use as needed when the symptoms include panic attacks. Also, during the period immediately following the traumatic event (i.e., ASD), benzodiazepines can be helpful for severe insomnia, particularly if due to traumatic nightmares, or for overwhelming anxiety. These recommendations are based on our clinical experience. The evidence for benzodiazepines is sparse and suggests that these agents may even have a negative impact if used chronically in PTSD. (For information regarding the individual benzodiazepines, including dosing and adverse reactions, see Chapter 7.)

KEY POINTS

- PTSD is difficult to recognize and diagnose because it "masquerades" as other disorders both medical and psychiatric.
- Over 80% of the time, PTSD is comorbid with another disorder (i.e., depression, substance abuse)
- To be considered a cause of PTSD, the traumatic event must be extreme (i.e., life-threatening) and produce feelings of being overwhelmed.
- The person needs to directly experience the traumatic event or witness it.
- Somatic symptoms are exceedingly common in PTSD.
- Use an individualized treatment approach combining psychotherapy and medications.
- An experienced psychotherapist is more important than the type of psychotherapy.
- Antidepressants, particularly SSRIs, are the backbone of pharmacotherapy in PTSD.
- Other agents—particularly trazodone, atypical antipsychotics, and antiepileptic drugs—are effectively used in combination with an antidepressant for some patients with PTSD.

REFERENCES

1. McFarlane AC, Atchison E, Rafaloxicz E, et al. Physical symptoms in post-traumatic stress disorder. *J Pyschosom Res.* 1994;38:715-26.
2. Shalev AY. What is post-traumatic stress disorder? *J Clin Psychiatry.* 2001; 62(suppl 17):4-10.
3. Goldstein G, van Kammen W, Shelly C, et al. Survivors of imprisonment in the Pacific theater during World War II. *Am J Psychiatry.* 1987;144:1210-1213.
4. Liebschutz J, Saitz R, Brower V, et al. PTSD in urban primary care: high prevalence and low physician recognition. *J Gen Intern Med.* 2007;22(6):719-726.

KEY REFERENCES

American Psychiatric Association. Practice guidelines for the treatment of patients with acute stress disorder and posttraumatic stress disorder. *Am J Psychiatry.* 2004;161:3-31.

Ballenger JC, Davidson JR, Lecrubier Y, et al. Consensus statement on posttraumatic stress disorder from the International Consensus Group on Depression and Anxiety. *J Clin Psychiatry.* 2000;61:60-66.

Cooper J, Carty J, Creamer M. Pharmacotherapy for posttraumatic stress disorder: empirical review and clinical recommendations. *Aust NZ J Psychiatry.* 2005; 39(8):674-682.

Davis LL, English BA, Ambrose SM, et al. Pharmacotherapy for post-traumatic stress disorder: a comprehensive review. *Expert Opin Pharmacother.* 2001;2(10):1583-1595.

Iancu I, Rosen Y, Moshe K. Antiepileptic drugs in posttraumatic stress disorder. *Clin Neuropharmacol.* 2002;25(4):225-229.

Kessler RC, Borges B, Walters EE. Prevalence of and risk factors for lifetime suicide attempts in the National Comorbidity Survey. *Arch Gen Psychiatry.* 1999;56:617-626.

Nemeroff CB, Bremner JD, Foa EB, et al. Posttraumatic stress disorder: a state-of-the-science review. *J Psychiatr Res.* 2006;40(1):1-21.

North CS, Nixon SJ, Shariat S, et al. Psychiatric disorders among survivors of the Oklahoma City bombing. *JAMA.* 1999;282:755-762.

Robertson M, Humphreys L, Ray R. Psychological treatments for posttraumatic stress disorder: recommendations for the clinician based on a review of the literature. *J Psychiatr Pract.* 2004;10(2):106-118.

Stein DJ, Seedat S, van der Linden G, et al. Selective serotonin reuptake inhibitors in the treatment of post-traumatic stress disorder: a meta-analysis of randomized controlled trials. *International Clinical Psychopharmacology.* 2000;15:S31-S39.

Vieweg WV, Julius DA, Fernandez A, et al. Posttraumatic stress disorder: clinical features, pathophysiology, and treatment. *Am J Med.* 2006;119(5):383-390.

A

The Phobias

■ The Phobias and the General Clinician

A

"Ordinary" human fears include potentially dangerous or embarrassing circumstances. A phobia, on the other hand, is an irrational or objectively unfounded intense fear of an object or situation. Where and how to draw the line between "ordinary" human fears and phobias is somewhat arbitrary. The line is determined by the relationship between the intensity (i.e., discomfort) of the fear and the consequences (i.e., functional impairment) caused by the avoidance. In a clinically significant phobia, the anxiety is overwhelmingly intense. George Orwell depicted this terrifying experience in his book *1984*, in which the Ministry of Love used Winston's intense fear of rats (a specific phobia) to torture him in Room 101 to the point where he was "re-educated" and now "loved Big Brother." The severity of a phobia is determined in part by the proximity and frequency of the feared situation and by how much impairment results. For example, a needle phobia in a 19-year-old patient who is otherwise healthy is not nearly as significant as a needle phobia in a patient with end-stage renal disease requiring dialysis. The DSM-IV provides diagnostic criteria for specific phobias (i.e., simple phobias) and social phobia (i.e., social anxiety disorder), but it is the clinician's assessment that determines the degree of functional impairment.

When the phobic thoughts are long standing and pervasive (e.g., social phobia), patients restructure their entire lives in such a way to always avoid the phobic object or situation (also known as phobic avoidance). Elfriede Jelinek, the 2004 Nobel Prize winner in literature, responded to her invitation to Stockholm by saying: "I am not mentally able to withstand that. I have social phobia and cannot stand these large crowds of people." Whether patients with phobias will try to avoid the "torture" of confronting their phobia, like Winston in *1984*, or become handicapped or "tortured" by this very avoidance, like Jelinek, they live a life in abeyance. When phobias are recognized and diagnosed, especially earlier in life, effective treatment can put the person, rather than the phobia, back in charge and can prevent many of the life-altering consequences of unaddressed phobias.

In regard to the phobias, the general clinician's responsibilities are early recognition and diagnosis and appropriate management. The "essentials" required for these include an understanding of phobic avoidance as it pertains to specific phobias and social phobia; the diagnostic criteria for specific phobias and social phobia; screening questions and strategies to diagnose specific phobias and social phobia; and the tools for management of phobias, particularly exposure therapies and the role of medication.

■ Essential Terms and Concepts

Phobic Avoidance

The behaviors that people use to avoid contact with the feared entity (e.g., person, animal, place, thing, or situation) are referred to as "phobic avoidance." Phobic avoidance is the central feature in specific phobias and social phobia, but it can also occur in agoraphobia accompanying panic disorder and post-traumatic stress disorder (PTSD). In agoraphobia, the person avoids places that are difficult to escape from if a panic attack occurs; in PTSD, the person avoids any triggers that promote re-experiencing of the traumatic event. For social phobia, the phobic avoidance hinges on a fear of embarrassment or criticism that may occur in social settings. The phobic avoidance in specific phobias focuses on a particular object or situation. The phobic reaction and avoidance can generalize to stimuli associated with the object of the phobia (i.e., triggers). For example, some patients with health care related phobias develop conditioned avoidance of environmental triggers, such as the "smell of medicine," white coats, or the hospital environment in general, and will even avoid visiting family or friends who are hospitalized. In all cases of phobias, the person experiences significant distress and functional impairment from the phobic response itself. The measures he or she takes to avoid the phobic response (i.e., phobic avoidance) reduces the immediate distress of the phobic response, but in some cases, such avoidance may significantly restrict occupational or social functioning, which in turn results in emotional distress.

Specific Phobias

The symptoms of specific phobias are listed in Box 9-1.

The essential feature of specific phobias is fear or intense anxiety (including panic attacks) that is consistently provoked by a specific situation or object. Avoidance of the feared object or situation ensues. The DSM-IV divides specific phobias into 4 types: animal (e.g., spiders, snakes, dogs); natural environment (e.g., storms, heights, water); blood-injection or injury (e.g., medical or dental procedures); and situational (e.g., elevators, flying, public transportation). The diagnosis of

> **Box 9-1 Symptoms of Specific Phobias**
>
> - Dizziness and faintness
> - Palpitations
> - Abnormally rapid heartbeat
> - Sweating
> - Trembling
> - Nausea
> - Shortness of breath

specific phobias is only appropriate if symptoms cause marked distress and significant functional impairment (see Box 9-2).

The general clinician is most likely to see situational (e.g., fear of flying, performance anxiety) or blood-injection or injury subtypes. We will focus on the latter because they can significantly interfere with health care and are often not recognized. For some, even the thought of coming to the doctor's office or the hospital produces intense fear. Phobias of needles, the sight of blood or open wounds, pain, anesthesia, and dental procedures are all very common. The lifetime prevalence of phobias of blood, injections, or dentists is 3.5% with a median age of onset of 5.5 years. In clinical samples of patients with health care related phobias, fainting in the phobic situation is extremely common (up to 50%-75%); up to 75% of patients have experienced a characteristic vasovagal response (i.e., an accelerated heart rate followed by a deceleration in heart rate and a drop in blood pressure), usually in the doctor's office (1). While over half had told a clinician or other health care professional of their health care related fears, none reported seeking mental health treatment for their phobias.

> **Box 9-2 Specific Phobias: Criteria**
>
> - The person experiences a persistent and excessive fear of an object or situation that is cued by exposure to that object or situation.
> - Exposure provokes an intense anxiety response (i.e., a "fight-or-flight" response).
> - The person recognizes that the fear is unreasonable or irrational.
> - The phobic situation is avoided or endured with significant discomfort.
> - The above significantly interferes with the person's ability to function normally.

Social Phobia (Social Anxiety Disorder)

Social phobia often goes unrecognized and untreated. In the National Comorbidity Survey Replication Study (NCS-R), the median duration of delay of the first treatment was 16 years. Only 45% of people with social phobia in the community were receiving treatment, and over half of those receiving treatment were receiving it in a primary care setting. Adding to the complexity, over 80% of the time, social phobia co-occurs with another psychiatric disorder. Detecting social phobia and initiating treatment early in its course during young adulthood dramatically reduces the negative consequences caused by avoidance of social interactions and groups of people.

The essential feature of social phobia is a marked and persistent fear of social or performance situations in which embarrassment may occur (see Box 9-3). Patients with this condition are afraid that others will be critical of them and judge them to be stupid, inarticulate, weak, or "crazy." Fear of public speaking occurs both alone as performance anxiety (i.e., a specific phobia, situational subtype) and as part of the more pervasive disorder, social phobia. Performance anxiety is limited to public presentations, but

Box 9-3 Social Phobia (Social Anxiety Disorder): Criteria

- The person experiences a marked and persistent fear of social situations in which he or she is exposed to unfamiliar people.
- The person fears that he or she may act in a way that causes embarrassment.
- Exposure to these situations causes intense anxiety including panic attacks.
- The individual recognizes that the fears are irrational.
- The avoidance of the social situations interferes significantly with the person's normal routine, occupational functioning, or social relationships.

social phobia is more generalized and more debilitating because all interactions with other people are experienced essentially as "performances" that cause extreme discomfort. People with social phobia even experience extreme anxiety when anticipating conversation with others for fear that they will appear inarticulate or do something embarrassing. Many will not bring up these difficulties with their clinician because of embarrassment, so the general clinician must directly inquire. One common symptom in men with social phobia is fear of urinating in public restrooms to the point of inability to do so. Thus social phobia may first surface when the general clinician asks the patient to provide a urine sample.

Patients who have social phobia almost always experience symptoms of anxiety in the feared social situation. These symptoms include palpitations, tremors, sweating, gastrointestinal discomfort, diarrhea, muscle tension, blushing, and confusion. These symptoms often meet the criteria for a panic attack. Blushing, which is less common in other anxiety disorders, is typical of social phobia.

Epidemiology

According to the NCS-R, the lifetime prevalences of DSM-IV specific phobias and social phobia were 12.1% and 12.5%, respectively, making them the most common anxiety disorders found in the general population. The onset of symptoms for both phobias is in childhood; over half of the people with social phobia will have onset by age 13 (90% by age 23). Specific phobias typically have onset in childhood, too, but continue to develop throughout young adulthood. Women are generally more likely than men to have specific phobias, but this varies by subtype (e.g., 75%-90% of those with animal, situational, or natural environment subtypes are female; 55% of those with blood-injection or injury subtype are female). Women are about twice as likely as men to have social phobia, but men are more likely to seek treatment. As more women enter the workforce, assume performance roles, and find that social phobia symptoms interfere with their career success, it is likely that they will seek treatment at higher rates than at present.

Comorbidites

Both specific phobias and social phobia are highly comorbid with other psychiatric disorders. Patients with a specific phobia had 4 to 8 times the expected lifetime prevalence of other psychiatric conditions, including major depression, obsessive-compulsive disorder (OCD), panic disorder, agoraphobia, social phobia, and other simple phobias. Patients with social phobia have a comorbid disorder (e.g., depression, another anxiety disorder, substance abuse) present more than 80% of the time.

A

■ Case-Finding Strategies

Screening for Specific Phobias

The general clinician should consider screening for health care related phobias when a patient appears nervous without obvious reason, is unusually resistant to having a procedure or test, has an episode of fainting, has a high "no show" rate for appointments, or wants to leave the hospital against medical advice. In these situations, directly inquiring about the possibility of a phobic object or situation is most productive. Though we usually recommend against using jargon, most people know the word "phobia." The following are examples of good screening questions:

> *Do you think some kind of phobia is interfering with your coming to the office?*
>
> *What has happened in the past when you had _____?*
> *(e.g., blood collected, anesthesia, surgery)*
>
> *How have you managed these situations in the past?*

After exploring for phobias, the clinician should consider the possibility of other psychiatric disorders that may be comorbid. Finally, educating patients about effective treatments for phobias is usually calming for them and facilitates further discussion about management.

Screening Questions for Social Phobia

As noted earlier, patients with social phobia typically delay seeking treatment for many years after onset of symptoms—if they seek it all. These patients know something is wrong but attribute it to shortcomings in themselves. Their high level of embarrassment further inhibits them, so few would ever initiate discussion about this to a general clinician. Directly discussing social phobia with these patients is awkward because this inquiry can make the patient more self-conscious, irrationally confirm the patient's worries that "it shows," and make the anxiety and discomfort in the room palpable. Not infrequently, patients and clinicians collude and do not bring "it" up. However, using a direct, unambiguous, and sensitive approach can get both the patient and clinician through the major obstacle of initiating the discussion. The following questions can be useful:

Do you have this level of anxiety in other situations, too?

How long has it been like this?

Are you familiar with social phobia or social anxiety disorder?

Do you often fear being the center of attention?

Do you frequently fear you will embarrass yourself in public?

The first question distinguishes social phobia from specific phobias. The second question looks for the almost universal onset in childhood of social phobia. The last question serves to transition to the next part of the interview, in which the clinician establishes the diagnosis, explores comorbid conditions, and discusses management.

■ Treatment

Psychotherapy for Specific Phobias

Although they are extremely common, specific phobias do not often cause enough impairment to warrant extensive treatment. Many phobic patients are able to adapt their lifestyles in order to avoid contact with the feared stimulus without functional impairment. Many can navigate the infrequent exposure to the phobic object (e.g., flying, performing) with the aid of medications as needed (see Pharmacotherapy later in this chapter). However, if the patient's impairment becomes debilitating or interferes with significant activities—for example, a diabetic patient with a needle phobia—then the clinician should recommend a course of exposure-based treatment.

The treatment of specific phobias was an early focus of behavior therapy research. The effectiveness of exposure-based therapies has been well established in controlled trials. Exposure treatment involves gradual confrontation (i.e., exposure) with the phobic object. If the specific phobia is severe, then the therapist may only have the patient imagine the phobic object or situation. Depending on the level of the patient's anxiety response, the therapist finds a "distance" from the phobic object that the patient can tolerate (often only imagined) and from that point gradually approaches the phobic object until it is actually confronted in reality.

Exposure treatments when applied properly yield high success rates. It is very reasonable to expect a positive outcome in 75% to 90% of cases, and the benefits are maintained long term. Despite the availability of such effective treatments, only a small minority of people with specific phobias ever seek professional help.

These techniques are especially effective for patients with needle phobias who require medical procedures and for patients with flying phobias who must travel by airplane. It is important for these approaches to be applied by a skilled therapist, however, because exposure done prematurely or incorrectly can worsen the phobia.

Psychotherapy for Social Phobia

Like other anxiety disorders, social phobia can be effectively treated with psychotherapy. The studies testing drugs have mostly been short term and focused on symptom reduction. However, social phobia is a chronic condition, which can be debilitating in large measure because of the social impairment that is perpetuated by specific maladaptive behaviors and beliefs. At the core of social phobia are many misperceptions that distort social interactions. A patient with social phobia believes that others are highly critical of imperfect performance and can tell that the patient is anxious. Internally, the socially phobic patient views these criticisms as catastrophic. Psychotherapy plays a special and important role in the treatment of social phobia because it directly addresses management of the internal distress that arises in social settings; brings about (re)training of social skills; offers gradual guided exposure to feared social situations; and aids the patient in confronting his or her negative cognitions.

Cognitive behavioral therapy (CBT) that focuses on social retraining and guided exposure to social situations is very effective and more enduring than medications alone. Further, many of the maladaptive avoidant behaviors, sometimes called "safety behaviors," are maintained by the cognitive schemas previously mentioned (e.g., mistaken beliefs about being critically judged), even if medication has controlled overt manifestations of anxiety. CBT addresses symptoms, fears, and maladaptive thoughts and behaviors and allows the therapist and patient to tailor an individualized approach. Although combinations of psychotherapy and long-term treatment with medication have not been studied vigorously, most experts believe that such combinations are particularly effective in patients with social phobia, given the condition's chronic course and significant comorbidity. Without medication to control severe social anxiety, some patients will not be able to engage in psychotherapy, which after all is a form of social interaction in which patients are expected to express themselves and actively participate or "perform."

Pharmacotherapy

Specific phobias are typically not managed with medication long term. However, given their highly comorbid nature, chronic drug therapy may be indicated to treat a comorbid condition (most often depression or another anxiety disorder). Most of the medications for specific phobias (beta-blockers, benzodiazepines) are given on an as-needed basis. These as-needed medications are also helpful for social phobic patients, but sustained drug treatment plays a greater role for them.

Beta-blockers

The excessive sympathetic stimulation that frequently occurs with phobias produces somatic symptoms like sweating, increased heart rate, blushing, and tremor. These symptoms by themselves can cause significant distress, but in socially phobic patients they also trigger additional, escalating anxiety in the form of self-consciousness, embarrassment, and avoidant responses. Decreasing or preventing these physical symptoms with beta-blockers greatly reduces the distress caused in some phobic situations. However, while beta-blockers reduce peripheral adrenergic symptoms, they have little effect on central anxiety (i.e., the psychological experience of being nervous). Beta-blockers have been effectively used by students who suffer from test-taking phobias, by musicians and actors before performances, and by airplane passengers who suffer from situational travel phobia.

Agents with a short half-life (e.g., propranolol) are effective for presentations and performances. Most beta-blockers are effective. A test dose should be used before taking a beta-blocker during a "performance." Though side effects are infrequent, sedation, bradycardia, and hypotension may occur. Beta-blockers are useful for episodic, short-term use; studies have not supported their long-term use, and there are scarce data to support their use in treating social phobias.

Benzodiazepines

Benzodiazepines are also very effective in managing specific phobias. In contrast to beta-blockers, benzodiazepines reduce both central and peripheral manifestations of anxiety. For the person with a flying phobia who flies infrequently, a dose of a benzodiazepine before the flight may greatly reduce his or her distress. The use of a benzodiazepine before a concert performance may reduce the associated anxiety but may also interfere with peak performance if the musician becomes too relaxed. The possible side effects of sedation and short-term memory dysfunction can be counterproductive while taking a test or giving a presentation. If a benzodiazepine is used in these situations, a test dose at a noncrucial time is important to establish the patient's response and how it compares with the desired response.

Long-term use of benzodiazepines for specific phobias is not indicated. The available data suggest benzodiazepines (particularly clonazepam) are effective in reducing symptoms in patients with social phobia. However, there are little or no data on their long-term use in social phobia. We do not use a benzodiazepine as monotherapy for social phobia but may use one in combination with another agent (e.g., an antidepressant).

There is growing evidence that benzodiazepines may block the positive effects of exposure-based therapies. Apparently, if a phobic reaction is completely blocked with a benzodiazepine, the body does not respond in a way to extinguish future reactions. Therefore, benzodiazepines should usually be avoided while a patient is engaged in an exposure-based ther-apy. Benzodiazepines and their usage in generalized anxiety disorder (GAD) and panic disorder (PD) are discussed in more depth in Chapter 7.

Long-term Medications

As previously noted, there are no long-term medication treatments indi-cated for specific phobias; when a medication is used long term in a patient with a specific phobia, it is to treat a comorbid disorder.

A

Antidepressants are the backbone of pharmacotherapy for social pho-bia. In the last decade, selective serotonin reuptake inhibitors (SSRIs) and serotonin-norepinephrine reuptake inhibitors (SNRIs) have become the first-line agents for social phobia; SSRIs and SNRIs have a delayed onset of action and may paradoxically increase anxiety symptoms during the initial treatment period. In trials of SSRIs and SNRIs in social phobia for 8 to 12 weeks, response rates (not remission rates) typically range from 50% to 80%. When a sufficient response occurs, the clinician should continue drug therapy for at least 6 (and probably 12) months. As with the other anx-iety disorders, the clinician should start the antidepressant at half the usual starting dose and titrate up slowly. It may also be helpful to prescribe a low-dose benzodiazepine while initiating an SSRI or SNRI to help diminish anxiety-like side effects of the medication as well as to provide patients with particularly severe anxiety some immediate relief. Patients with social phobia have particular difficulty tolerating the mild tremor and excessive sweating, which are occasional side effects of SSRIs and SNRIs. (See Chap-ters 4 and 7 for more discussion, including dosing and adverse reactions.)

Fifteen published, randomized, double-blind, placebo-controlled trials of SSRIs in social anxiety disorder have shown them to be more effective than a placebo for social anxiety disorder, with improvement extending into social and occupational function (2). SNRIs (duloxetine and venlafaxine) are clinically used interchangeably with SSRIs, though neither carries an FDA-approved indication for social phobia.

Mirtazapine has 1 controlled trial supporting its use in social phobia and represents a good alternative if initial treatment with SSRIs fails or requires augmentation.

Monoamine oxidase inhibitors (MAOIs) are effective for social phobia but are typically only prescribed by psychiatrists in treatment-resistant cases. MAOIs were widely used for social phobia prior to SSRIs and are considered by some experts to still represent the "gold standard" in phar-macotherapy for social phobia. Side effects and drug and dietary restrictions limit their use today. When MAOIs are used, the general clinician needs to remember the dietary restrictions and significant potential drug interactions. (See Chapters 4 and 5 for more discussion, including adverse reactions and side effects.)

Gabapentin (Neurontin) and pregabalin (Lyrica) are both anticonvul-sants with similar chemical structures. Both have been studied in controlled trials in social phobia and have response rates better than a placebo. Gabapentin causes sedation and cognitive slowing in many patients and requires divided dosing. Typically, it is started at 100 mg at night and then gradually moved into daytime dosing. Ultimately, it is given in a total dose range of 900 to 3600 mg/day divided into 3 or 4 doses. Pregabalin was launched at the beginning of 2005 and only carries an FDA indication for the treatment of pain caused by diabetic neuropathy or herpetic neuralgia. Its use is limited by most managed pharmacy drug plans. Neither of these agents should be considered first-line or second-line treatments, but either may serve as an alternative or as an add-on therapy in treatment-resistant patients.

Buspirone (BuSpar) is not as potent as a monotherapy in social phobia. However, it may be used to augment another agent. Bupropion (Wellbutrin) is an effective monotherapy for depression but is not frequently used in the treatment of anxiety disorders, including social phobia. It is the most activating antidepressant and may paradoxically increase anxiety in some patients.

KEY POINTS

- A phobic reaction is an intense, automatic reaction that occurs when a person is confronted with a phobic object or situation.
- Phobic avoidance refers to the steps (i.e., "safety behaviors") taken by a phobic person to not confront the phobic object or situation or any stimuli associated with it.
- There are 4 types of specific phobias: animal, natural environment, blood-injection or injury, and situational.
- The general clinician is most likely to see health care related phobias in patients avoiding treatments or procedures.
- Because of embarrassment, people with phobias seldom discuss them, so direct questions are required.
- Specific phobias are effectively treated with exposure-based therapies.
- Social phobia is a pervasive fear of embarrassment or criticism in a social situation.
- A mean duration of 16 years occurs between onset of symptoms and treatment in social phobia.
- Phobias start in childhood; over 90% of patients with social phobia have onset before age 23.
- Social phobia is comorbid with another disorder 80% of the time.
- Early detection and treatment reduces lifetime morbidity of avoidance behaviors.
- CBT is very effective in long-term management of social phobia.

References

1. Bienvenu OJ, Eaton WW. The epidemiology of blood-injection-injury phobia. *Psychological Medicine.* 1998;28:1129-1136.
2. Hedges DW, Brown BL, Shwalb DA, et al. The efficacy of selective serotonin reuptake inhibitors in adult social anxiety disorder: a meta-analysis of double-blind, placebo-controlled trials. *J Psychopharmacol.* 2007;21:102-111.

Key References

Antony MM, Swinson RP. *Phobic Disorders and Panic in Adults: A Guide to Assessment and Treatment.* Washington, DC: American Psychological Association; 2000.

Jefferson JW. Benzodiazepines and anticonvulsants for social phobia (social anxiety disorder). *J Clin Psychiatry.* 2001;62(1):50-53.

Kessler RC, Berglund P, Demler O, et al. Lifetime prevalence and age-of-onset distributions of DSM-IV disorders in the National Comorbidity Survey Replication. *Arch Gen Psychiatry.* 2005;65:593-602.

Stein MB. An epidemiologic perspective on social anxiety disorder. *J Clin Psychiatry.* 2006;67:3-8.

Schneier FR. Social Anxiety Disorder. *New Engl J Med.* 2006;355:1029-1036.

Versiani M. A review of 19 double-blind placebo-controlled studies in social anxiety disorder (social phobia). *World J Biol Psychiatry.* 2000;1(1):27-33.

A

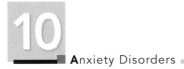

Obsessive-Compulsive Disorder

■ Obsessive-Compulsive Disorder and the General Clinician

A

In the movie *As Good As It Gets*, Melvin Udall (played by Jack Nicholson) methodically washes his hands 3 times with 3 different, individually wrapped bars of soap, can barely walk down a sidewalk for fear of stepping on a crack, locks the door 5 times, and turns the lights on and off 5 times. This character captures many of the core features of obsessive-compulsive disorder (OCD) and conveys the isolation and shame associated with the disorder.

Understanding the shame and isolation associated with OCD helps us understand why people suffering with OCD rarely reveal it to their treating clinicians. Though over two-thirds of people with OCD have their onset of symptoms before age 15 years, most do not present for treatment until after age 27 years.

OCD is similar to social phobia in that both have an early onset, long delay in seeking treatment, and considerable associated shame and embarrassment. The general clinician's responsibilities are also similar in both cases: first, to recognize the disorder early in its course and diagnosis it properly, then to appropriately facilitate management of the disorder to prevent long-term sequelae. The "essentials" required include understanding obsessions and compulsions, the diagnostic criteria for OCD, screening questions and techniques, and management strategies.

■ Essential Concepts and Terms

Obsessions and Compulsions

Either obsessions or compulsions are required for the diagnosis of OCD, but both obsessions and compulsions appear in greater than 80% of cases of OCD (1). Obsessions are defined as persistent ideas, thoughts, impulses, or images that feel intrusive, uncontrollable, and inappropriate. *Obsessions increase anxiety.* The patient will often attempt to ignore, suppress, neutralize, or undo these obsessions with some other thought or action (i.e., compulsions). *Compulsions reduce anxiety.* Compulsions are repetitive behaviors (e.g., rituals) or mental acts that are aimed at preventing or

Box 10-1 Obsessions and Compulsions Defined

Obsessive-compulsive disorder includes either *obsessions* or *compulsions* with subsequent marked functional impairment.

- *Obsessions*: Increase anxiety. Recurrent and persistent thoughts, impulses, or images that are excessive and feel bad.
- *Compulsions*: Decrease anxiety. Repetitive behaviors or mental acts that the person feels driven to do in response to the obsession that are recognized as excessive.

alleviating the anxiety and distress caused by the obsessions (see Box 10-1).

Frequently, particular obsessions couple with specific sets of compulsions. When one half of the "coupling" is identified (e.g., hand washing), then the other half (e.g., fear of contamination with germs) is directly pursued. Nicholson's Melvin Udall had the common pairing of the obsessional fear of contamination with germs and the compulsion to wash or clean; the fear of contamination increases his anxiety, and the cleaning and washing reduce it. Another common coupling is an obsessional fear of disorder with a compulsion to establish order or symmetry through rearrangement. In this case, a stack of magazines can serve as the stimulus for obsessions about whether to order them by size, shape, color, and so on. If the patient is in a public place, and rearranging the magazines will attract a lot of attention, then a less conspicuous compulsion of counting ordered series of numbers (e.g., by twos, by primes, by multiples) may be used to reduce the obsession. At such a person's home, the need for a highly ordered living space may result in hours spent daily rearranging and maintaining elaborate systems of organization. Any disruption in the order of things is intolerable. Obsessional fears of intruders or fires are frequently coupled with compulsive repetitive checking that doors and windows are locked or stoves and toasters are turned off.

People suffering from OCD are more than very neat or orderly people. In common parlance, people may be referred to as "compulsive" or "anal" when they are very particular about certain things, like their cars or their clothes. These individuals have perfectionistic personality traits, and while they can also have OCD, they usually do not. In OCD the obsessions and compulsions have 4 essential features:

1. The obsessions cause severe internal distress, as does not being able to carry out the compulsions.
2. The activities are recognized by the patient as excessive and irrational.
3. Over 1 hour per day (typically more) is consumed with these activities.
4. The activities interfere with relationships.

Epidemiology

The best estimate is that about 2.2% of Americans will develop OCD in their lifetimes. OCD seems to affect men and women about equally. Men typically have an earlier age of onset (6 to 15 years) than women (20 to 30 years) (2).

Comorbidities

OCD is highly comorbid with other psychiatric disorders. In the Brown Longitudinal Obsessive Compulsive Study, the lifetime comorbity for another psychiatric disorder was 91%. Table 10-1 gives the lifetime comorbidity rates for the most common comorbid disorders (1).

Trichotillomania

The lifetime prevalence rates of trichotillomania for college-aged men and women are 1.3% and 3.4%, respectively, with onset usually in childhood or adolescence (3). Pulling or twisting the hair from either one's scalp or eyelashes is most frequent. Women present for treatment more frequently, but men's secondary hair loss to trichotillomania is not as apparent and thus reduces their impetus for treatment. Pharmacologic and psychotherapeutic treatment approaches are similar to those for OCD (see Treatment later in this chapter).

Tourette Syndrome

About one-half of people with tourette syndrome (TS) have OCD, and as already mentioned, about 10% of people with OCD have TS. TS is a neurobiological disorder characterized by involuntary muscle movements (i.e., tics) and vocal outbursts that are often disruptive. There is a misperception that the vocal utterances are profane, but fewer than 15% of the vocal utterances are cursing, obscenities, or racial slurs. Many patients with TS do not require treatment for the management of their tics. The agents used when treatment is required include typical antipsychotics (e.g., haloperidol, fluphenazine); atypical antipsychotics (e.g., risperidone, olanzapine); clonidine; and benzodiazepines (e.g., clonazepam). OCD combined with TS is

Table 10-1 Lifetime Comorbidity Rates for OCD and the Most Common Comorbid Disorders

Any mood disorder	75%
Any anxiety disorder	53%
Any substance abuse disorder	26%
Any eating disorder	10%
Any tic disorder (e.g., Tourette syndrome)	14%
Any impulse control disorder (e.g., trichotillomania)	15%

usually managed with a selective serotonin reuptake inhibitor (SSRI) first. Antipsychotics, clonidine, or bennzodiazepines can be added if needed. Psychotherapies are extremely important for long-term management.

■ Case-Finding Strategies

OCD is considered a "hidden" disease by some because it is frequently undiagnosed. The shame and embarrassment of patients with OCD compels them to conceal their compulsions or obsessions. Patients with OCD may be willing to report "anxiety" or "depression" but are reluctant to volunteer their obsessions and compulsions.

To find out if obsessions and compulsions are present, the clinician must inquire directly. Mentioning common obsession-compulsion pairings as examples cues the patient with OCD that you "know about OCD." One of our patients recently volunteered, "I was so relieved when you asked me how many times I washed my plate before using it, because it let me know that you knew what 'this' was and that I was not crazy." This patient was 52 years old and had been treated for depression for the last 8 years without recognition of her OCD, which had started in her early 20s.

For the general clinician, the most common situation in which screening for OCD occurs is after he or she diagnoses one psychiatric disorder (e.g., depression) and then assesses for a possible second (i.e., co-morbid) psychiatric disorder. Direct, clear screening questions, similar in style to questions used when screening for phobias, are best:

> *Do you have any thoughts or rituals that interfere with your regular activities?*

If the patient does not respond immediately or seems hesitant, add some examples:

> *I'm asking about thoughts or rituals like repeatedly washing your hands, counting particular sequences of numbers over and over, or going back to check the house's door lock several times even though you know it is locked.*

If they acknowledge having uncomfortable obsessions, inquire how they manage or cope with them and how much time each day is spent in these activities. Also ask when these symptoms started, because frequently the symptoms predate the "presenting" psychiatric disorder.

■ Treatment

Psychotherapy

Psychotherapy, particularly cognitive behavioral therapy (CBT), is at least as effective as pharmacotherapy in OCD. CBT has virtually no side effects, and when administered by a good psychotherapist, it produces therapeutic gains that are maintained over long-term follow-up. The CBT used in OCD is similar to the exposure-based therapies for specific phobias and social phobia. The behavioral therapy for OCD involves exposure and response prevention (ERP), which is based on the fact that anxiety diminishes with repeated contact with the feared object. ERP has to go a step further in OCD than the exposure therapies for phobias because the person's ritualized response to the fear has to be addressed, too. For example, an OCD patient with a contamination obsession and a hand washing compulsion may be asked to imagine and eventually touch something dirty (e.g., the floor, a doorknob) and then resist washing his or her hands. The longer he or she can resist, the better. Homework includes practicing at home and logging the experiences.

The cognitive component is added to the therapy to confront the exaggerated or catastrophic thing that often accompanies the obsession-compulsion couplings. For example, "If I do not wash my hands, then I'll get an infection and then that may spread and then I'll die." These automatic thoughts or irrational cognitive schemas are similar to the social phobic ideas of presumed expectations of perfection and exaggerated criticisms by others.

Pharmacotherapy

Antidepressants are the mainstay of pharmacotherapy for OCD. In the last decade SSRIs and SNRIs have become the first-line agents for OCD. However, SSRIs and serotonin-norepinephrine reuptake inhibitors (SNRIs) have a delayed onset of action and may paradoxically increase anxiety symptoms during the initial treatment period. Not all of these agents carry approval from the FDA for the treatment of OCD, but we consider all SSRIs and SNRIs appropriate choices for OCD. As with the other anxiety disorders, medications should be started at half of the usual starting dose and titrated up slowly.

It may also be helpful to prescribe a low-dose benzodiazepine while initiating an SSRI or SNRI to help diminish anxiety-like side effects of the medication as well as to provide some immediate relief if the patient is having significant acute anxiety.

Fluvoxamine (i.e., Luvox, Luvox CR) has been portrayed as unique among the SSRIs for treatment of OCD. Though it was the first SSRI to carry FDA approval for OCD, it is similar in efficacy and side effects to the other SSRIs. We rarely use fluvoxamine because it has the highest likelihood among the SSRIs of drug-drug interactions. See Chapters 4 and 7 for more discussion, including dosing and adverse reactions of all the SSRIs and SNRIs.

SNRIs such as duloxetine and venlafaxine are used interchangeably with SSRIs, though neither carries an FDA-approved indication for OCD. While case reports and double-blind studies comparing SNRIs to other drugs in OCD support their efficacy, placebo-controlled studies with venlafaxine and duloxetine have not yet been reported. We consider both agents reasonable choices for the treatment of OCD.

Tricyclic antidepressants (TCAs) and especially clomipramine (Anafranil) are also effective in the treatment of OCD. Clomipramine was a breakthrough drug when it was released in the United States in 1989, already widely used in Europe and Canada. Clomipramine was the most serotonergic TCA and provided relief for many patients with OCD until the introduction of SSRIs in the 1990s. A large number of placebo-controlled and active comparison trials with clomipramine document its efficacy in OCD, and meta-analytic studies suggest a small superiority over SSRIs, but its strong anticholinergic side effects have relegated it to use as an alternative when SSRIs fail or are not tolerated (4). Patients are more likely to be able to develop tolerance of its side effects with the "start low, go slow" approach to dosage.

Benzodiazepines help some patients with OCD to manage acute anxiety or exacerbation of symptoms but are not effective as a monotherapy. As noted in Chapter 9, there is growing evidence the benzodiazepines may interfere with the lasting effects of exposure-based psychotherapies. We recommend reviewing this with the psychotherapist who is conducting the CBT before prescribing a benzodiazepine. Otherwise these agents are very effective in reducing periodic escalations of anxiety.

Atypical antipsychotics have an emerging role for refractory or difficult-to-treat OCD. These agents should be considered when the symptoms remain intrusive and functional impairment is high despite maximized antidepressant dosage. As previously noted, these agents are effective in trichotillomania and TS and work well in combination with most SSRIs when OCD is comorbid with these disorders.

KEY POINTS

- Obsessions increase anxiety. Obsessions are recurrent and persistent thoughts, impulses, or images that are excessive and feel bad.
- Compulsions decrease anxiety. Compulsions are repetitive behaviors or mental acts that the person feels driven to do in response to the obsession, and he or she recognizes them as excessive.

- Patients are often ashamed and secretive about their obsessions and compulsions and do not usually volunteer information unless directly asked.
- Depressive disorders co-occur with OCD up to 80% of the time.
- About one-half of people with TS have OCD, and 15% of patients with OCD have TS.
- Trichotillomania occurs in 10% to 15% of patients with OCD.
- SSRIs are the drug class of choice in treating OCD.
- CBT is highly effective in treating OCD.
- Exposure response prevention is the recommended behavioral component of CBT for patients with OCD.

A

REFERENCES

1. Pinto A, Mancebo MC, Eisen JL, et al. The Brown Longitudinal Obsessive Compulsive Study: clinical features and symptoms of the sample at intake. *J Clin Psychiatry.* 2006;67:703-711.
2. Office of the Surgeon General. Mental Health: A Report of the Surgeon General. Dec 13, 1999. Available at: http://www.surgeongeneral.gov/library/mentalhealth/home.html. Accessed August 17, 2007.
3. Ko SM. Under-diagnosed psychiatric syndrome I: trichotillomania. *Ann Acad Med Singap.* 1999; 28(2):279-81.
4. Denys D. Pharmacotherapy of obsessive-compulsive disorder and obsessive-compulsive spectrum disorders. *Psychiatr Clin North Am.* 2006;29(2):553-584.

KEY REFERENCES

Blier P, Habib R, Flament MF. Pharmacotherapies in the management of obsessive-compulsive disorder. *Can J Psychiatry.* 2006;51(7):417-430.

Dell'Osso B, Nestadt G, Allen A, et al. Serotonin-norepinephrine reuptake inhibitors in the treatment of obsessive-compulsive disorder: a critical review. *J Clin Psychiatry.* 2006;67(4):600-610.

Goodman WK, Storch EA, Geffken GR, et al. Obsessive-compulsive disorder in Tourette syndrome. *J Child Neurol.* 2006;21(8):704-714.

Heyman I, Mataix-Cols D, Fineberg NA. Obsessive-compulsive disorder. *BMJ.* 2006; 333(7565):424-429.

Nestadt G, Bienvenu OJ, Cai G, et al. Incidence of obsessive-compulsive disorder in adults. *J Nerv Ment Dis.* 1998;186:401-406.

Neziroglu F, Henricksen J, Yaryura-Tobias JA. Psychotherapy of obsessive-compulsive disorder and spectrum: established facts and advances, 1995-2005. *Psychiatr Clin North Am.* 2006;29(2):585-604.

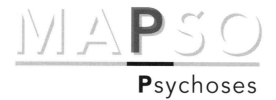

Psychoses

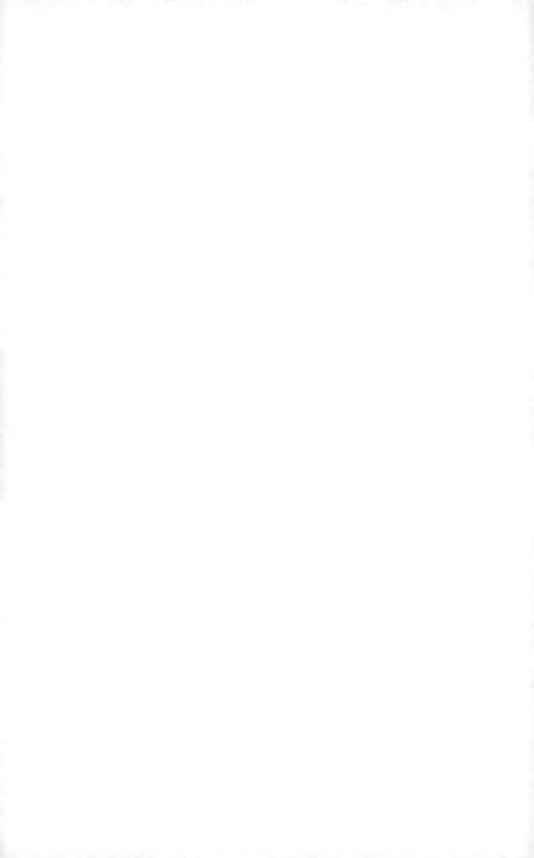

The Psychoses

■ The "Psychoses" and the General Clinician

Typically, a clinician will only consider a diagnosis of schizophrenia when encountering a patient with psychotic symptoms, but many psychiatric disorders present with psychotic symptoms. While mood disorders predominantly present with a mood disturbance (e.g., depression, mania), psychotic symptoms can also be present. Similarly, psychotic disorders predominantly present with psychosis (e.g., schizophrenia), but a mood disturbance can also be present. The key point is to not assume that all patients with psychotic symptoms have schizophrenia.

DSM-IV nosology contributes to the confusion by using the diagnostic category "psychotic disorders" to refer *only* to psychiatric disorders in which psychotic symptoms are *most* prominent and characteristic (e.g., schizophrenia) and not to *all* disorders in which psychosis can occur regardless of whether it is the most prominent symptom or not (e.g., bipolar I, psychotic depression). We entitled this chapter "The Psychoses" in an effort to address the confusing DSM-IV nosology, and we include discussion of *all* psychiatric disorders that may have psychosis as part of their presentation.

In keeping with the purpose of this book, we approach the discussion on psychosis from a primary care clinical perspective; that is, we start with affective disorders that can have psychotic symptoms that are more frequently seen in the primary care setting and then proceed to discuss schizophrenia, the most common psychotic disorder, which affects about 1% of the general population. In the past, primary care clinicians have not typically managed patients with schizophrenia, but recently an increasing number of nonpsychiatric clinicians have become the primary providers for schizophrenic patients, including writing prescriptions for their antipsychotic medications. In this chapter we cover both the general clinicians' role in recognizing and treating "nonschizophrenic" disorders that can present with psychotic symptoms as well as the challenges in managing antipsychotic treatment and medical treatment for schizophrenic patients. While we believe that patients with schizophrenia and other serious mental disorders with psychotic symptoms should have psychiatrists managing their care, we recognize the realities of the shortage and geographic maldistribution of psychiatrists, which means that the management of these patients is often left in the hands of general clinicians. The "essential" information and skills in this chapter include discussion of nonpsychotic disorders that occur in the primary care setting in which psychosis is present or should be considered (see Box 11-1). We also discuss "mimics" and screening strategies for uncovering possible past psychotic episodes. The chapter concludes with a discussion of schizophrenia and a detailed review of antipsychotic medications. Even if a psychiatrist is prescribing the antipsychotic medication, other clinicians following the patient should be familiar with the potential adverse medical effects of antipsychotics.

Box 11-1 Differential Diagnosis of Psychotic Symptoms

Paranormal experiences
Affective disorders
    Psychotic depression
    Bipolar I: mania with psychosis
Organic disorders
    Medical mimics
    Delirium
    Dementia
    Substance-induced psychosis
        Intoxication
        Withdrawal
Psychiatric mimics
    PTSD and borderline personality disorder
    Psychotic disorders
        Schizophrenia
        Schizoaffective disorder
        Delusional disorder

■ Essential Concepts and Terms

Psychosis

> *Doctor, I'm a doctor now too, and I can diagnose any illness just by looking at someone, and curing them by laying on of my hands.*

> *Doctor, I know my body is full of cancer, I'm going blind, and my liver is already dead, and this is punishment from God for my terrible sins.*

> *There are tiny robot bugs that invade my body at night and are controlled by my neighbor, who is a devil.*

Each of these statements is an example of psychosis, and each is from a different psychiatric disorder (respectively mania, psychotic depression, and schizophrenia). Psychosis is an internal, personal experience that is perceived as real by a psychotic individual and, by definition, is not regarded as real by others. Psychotic individuals incorrectly evaluate the accuracy of their perceptions and thoughts and make incorrect inferences about the external world even when faced with inarguable, contrary evidence. This incorrect set of perceptions and beliefs is called impaired reality testing. Psychotic individuals cannot effectively test their realities because 3 specific features of psychosis interfere: abnormal perceptions (hallucinations), fixed false beliefs (delusions), and disorganized thought processes.

Hallucinations

Hallucinations can involve any of the 5 senses: auditory, visual, tactile, olfactory, and gustatory. Auditory hallucinations are the most common form of hallucinations in psychiatric disorders but can occur in medical conditions also. Typically, a hallucinating patient hears a discernable voice. Sometimes he or she hears a noise (e.g., music) or a group of voices. These voices or sounds are different from the individual's own voice or sounds in his or her environment. The clinician should inquire about what the voices are saying, especially in the case of command hallucinations (see the screening questions later in this chapter).

Visual hallucinations do occur in psychotic affective disorders and schizophrenia, but they are much more suggestive of an organic cause. Delirium frequently presents with psychotic symptoms, including visual hallucinations. In the hospital, it is not uncommon to see a patient with delirium staring at some imagined thing in the air or picking at some imagined thing on the sheets. Visual hallucinations of terrifying animals are common in delirium tremens and other extreme withdrawal states.

Tactile, olfactory, and gustatory hallucinations are primarily associated with organic etiologies. Tactile hallucinations can occur in alcohol and sedative-hypnotic withdrawal states (e.g., formication). Olfactory hallucinations are commonly associated with temporal lobe epilepsy, particularly as an aura of the smell of burning rubber or other pungent smell before a seizure, and with CNS tumors. Gustatory hallucinations are the least common and can also be an aura manifestation in temporal lobe epilepsy.

Not all hallucinations are pathological. Hypnogogic and hypnopompic hallucinations are the vivid, fleeting hallucinations many normal people experience as they are going to sleep or waking up. They are also a common feature in narcolepsy. In acute grief, it is not unusual for the bereaved to see or hear the deceased during the first few weeks of grieving (see Chapter 3). Hallucinations also occur in some religious or spiritual states of mind (e.g., trance, ecstasy, meditation, communing with the spirit). All of these can occur without indicating mental illness.

Delusions

Delusions are fixed false beliefs that are not consistent with one's culture or religion. Common delusions include the following:

- Delusions of reference: The patient perceives that there are special messages from the TV, newspaper, or radio being directed to him or her.
- Delusions of persecution: The patient believes that agencies, certain individuals, or strangers are "out to get him or her" or are following him or her.
- Delusions of mind-reading: The patient believes that he or she can read minds or that others can read his or her mind.

■ Thought broadcasting: Related to delusions of mind-reading, the patient believes others can hear his or her thoughts as if they were out loud.

■ Delusions of thought control: The patient believes that others can control his or her thoughts, including inserting or withdrawing thoughts.

■ Delusions of grandiosity: The patient believes that he or she has amazing accomplishments and great powers, even godlike ones. This symptom strongly suggests mania.

■ Somatic delusions: For example, the patient believes she is pregnant or is riddled with cancer or a part of the body is under the control of some force outside the individual.

Delusions in schizophrenia are usually very bizarre (like the example of the robot bugs), while in affective disorders they tend to reflect the patient's predominant mood. The patient who believes he or she is a doctor with special medical powers is demonstrating the grandiosity and elation of mania, while the patient who believes his or her body is diseased as punishment for sin is expressing the guilt and negativism of severe psychotic depression.

Symptoms of Disorganization

Symptoms of disorganization include thought disorder, confusion, disconnection between thoughts and actions, and memory problems. This set of symptoms is associated with severe psychotic disorders, particularly schizophrenia. Symptoms of disorganized thoughts typically present during an acute exacerbation of the psychotic disorder, though some patients suffer from chronic disorganization. Speech that is easily derailed or incoherent, odd behaviors and movements that appear to have no purpose, or thoughts that do not seem connected to each other are all examples of disorganization.

Paranormal Experiences

Most of us have had experiences that leave us feeling odd or experiences that are outside of our culture's collective experience. These include experiences of déjà vu, premonitions, superstitions, and even belief in phenomena like extrasensory perception and telepathy. Paranormal experiences that are not caused by a disorder do not cause dysfunction, are limited in scope, are not bizarre, and are not considered delusions.

Psychotic Disorders

Psychotic disorders (e.g., schizophrenia, schizoaffective disorder, delusional disorder) are grouped together in this category because they all have psychotic symptoms as the predominant aspect of their presentations. This grouping also facilitates the creation of differential diagnoses of psychotic symptoms (e.g., substance-induced psychosis, delirium, dementia).

"Organic" psychoses are subsequently discussed, followed by a review of schizophrenia. Delirium and dementia are discussed in Chapter 13.

Organic Psychoses

Medical (Secondary) Causes of Psychosis

The distinction between delirium and psychotic symptoms that are caused by a medical condition or substance is one of degree. Delirium (see Chapter 13) is an encephalopathy diffusely affecting the brain. Psychotic symptoms frequently occur in delirium. One review of 227 consecutive patients with delirium found that 42.7% had at least one psychotic symptom. Visual hallucinations (27%) were most frequently observed. An altered sensorium and level of consciousness (e.g., hyperalert, somnolent), disorientation, and cognitive dysfunction usually distinguish delirium from the other psychoses (1).

There are many medical conditions that may cause one or many psychotic symptoms with or without delirium, particularly focal CNS lesions (e.g., tumor, stroke, vasculitis), CNS infections, CNS degenerative disorders, severe metabolic disturbances or endocrinopathies, and psychomotor seizures (see Box 11-2). For a full review and more complete list, see Masand et al (2).

> **Box 11-2 Examples of Medical (Secondary) Causes of Psychosis**
>
> Vitamin B deficiencies (e.g., thiamine, B12)
> Hyponatremia
> Hepatic encephalopathy
> Uremia
> CNS tumor
> Stroke
> HIV encephalopathy
> Encephalitis
> CNS vasculitis
> Wilson disease
> Huntington disease
> Psychomotor seizures

Substance-induced Psychosis

Cocaine and amphetamine intoxication both cause psychosis that can be acutely indistinguishable from psychosis caused by schizophrenia or depression. Substance-induced psychosis is typically acute and short-lived in a young adult. Other agents such as PCP, LSD, other hallucinogens, and newer "club drugs" (e.g., ecstasy) can all cause psychosis, too. Note that many hallucinogens and most of the newer club drugs are not included in a routine toxicology screen and should be specifically requested if suspected. Psychosis is also a symptom of withdrawal from alcohol and sedative-hypnotics. Chronic abuse of alcohol combined with poor nutrition causes alcoholic hallucinosis, which is neither intoxication nor a withdrawal state. The list of medications that can cause delirium and psychosis is vast. Chapter 13 discusses delirium in detail. One of the first steps when evaluating a patient with psychotic symptoms is to review the list of medications the patient is taking.

The list of all potential agents is too long to include here, but anticholinergic drugs, corticosteroids, and opioids are the most common causes

Box 11-3 Examples of Medications That Can Induce Psychosis

Antiarrhythmics
Anticholinergics
Antidepressants
Antihistamines
Antimalarials
Antivirals
Ciprofloxacin
Corticosteroids
Dopamine agonists
Opioids
Sympathomimetics

of medication-induced psychosis (see Box 11-3). Substance-induced disorders in general are more fully discussed in Chapter 12.

Psychiatric Mimics

Occasionally, symptoms in some other psychiatric disorders may be mistaken for psychosis. Patients with PTSD may have sensory experiences so vivid that they seem to be part of psychosis. For example, a patient reported periodically hearing organ music. It was not accompanied by other psychotic symptoms or depression, but it led to increased anxiety that she associated with her flashbacks. She later recalled that organ music had played while she was raped in a choir loft at church. Dissociative states, seen in severe cases of PTSD (see Chapter 8), can appear psychotic in their sometimes bizarre presentations but in fact represent some form of re-experience. Patients typically do not recall these events after they return to their "normal" states.

Patients with borderline personality disorder can have episodes of transient psychosis when under stress. The psychosis is typically experienced as paranoia or as auditory or visual hallucinations and resolves as the stressor passes. Patients with paranoid personality disorder by definition are suspicious and feel mistreated, but their paranoia usually remains in the realm of the possible. The behavior of those with schizotypal personality disorder often appears odd and even bizarre, and they may have unrealistic beliefs. In reality, the boundaries between these conditions and psychotic disorders can be blurry. The basic difference is one of degree, but disorganized behavior and the extent of loss of touch with reality also separate psychotic disorders from these personality disorders. (See Chapter 15 for further discussion.)

The Affective Psychoses

Psychotic Depression (Major Depressive Disorder with Psychotic Features)

Psychotic features can occur in up to 15% of depressed patients. Auditory hallucinations are the most commonly found psychotic symptoms. Feelings of extreme worthlessness or excessive guilt can be a good indicator of the possible presence of psychotic features.

Psychotic depression can occur at all ages, but when it occurs in young people, it strongly suggests that the patient will eventually turn out to have bipolar disorder. In a large naturalistic study of young adults (average age 23), 80% of those admitted with psychotic depression developed bipolar disorder in the subsequent 15 years (3). New onset of psychotic depression in the elderly may be the beginning of dementia.

All patients with major depression should be screened for psychosis even if no symptoms are evident or reported (see Screening Psychosis section). Often the psychotic symptoms include self-deprecating voices, delusional guilt, or obsessional hypochondriasis that reaches delusional proportions. In severe cases, some patients with psychotic depression experience auditory hallucinations that command the patient to take action. Command hallucinations to kill oneself constitute an emergency and require psychiatric hospitalization. Rates of completed suicide during an episode of psychotic depression are among the highest. Initial treatment includes an antidepressant plus an antipsychotic, but the most effective treatment for severe psychotic depression is electroconvulsive therapy (ECT), which is sometimes required on an emergent basis. Antipsychotics may not be required long term in psychotic, unipolar depression. Usually one is continued for about 6 months after the depression and psychotic symptoms resolve and then discontinued, whereas the antidepressant is continued chronically.

Bipolar I—Manic Episode with Psychosis

Psychosis can be present in either a manic or mixed episode in bipolar I disorder. Psychotic mania has been frequently misdiagnosed as schizophrenia, but the longitudinal course usually differentiates these 2 disorders. Delirium and mania share several symptoms (e.g., psychosis, poor sleep, and agitation), but delirium includes clouding of consciousness and cognitive dysfunction, which mania does not, and delirium mostly occurs in the context of severe medical illness. Mania with psychosis is an emergency requiring psychiatric hospitalization. Impulsivity and mood lability in mania combined with the delusions of psychosis can be very dangerous, with risk of suicide or harm to others. Treatment includes prescribing an antipsychotic until a mood stabilizer can take effect. ECT is very effective in mania and is the treatment of choice in extreme mania.

Dementia

Psychotic symptoms are common in most dementias (especially Alzheimer disease and Lewy body dementia). Delusions and hallucinations occur in 36% and 18%, respectively, of patients with Alzheimer dementia. Taking a careful history with the caregiver present is most productive in these situations. The dementias are reviewed in Chapter 13.

■ Case-Finding Strategies

Evaluating Psychotic Symptoms

The general clinician should be able to assess psychotic symptoms. Most often this will be part of gathering past psychiatric history in a patient who is not presently psychotic but who requires an assessment for a past history of psychosis—for example, in a patient with depression or bipolar disorder before starting a medication. Clinicians should also be prepared to evaluate the extent of psychosis in a patient suspected to be currently psychotic.

Screening for Psychosis

Discussing the possibility of psychosis with patients is tricky. Asking about hallucinations and delusions often elicits defensive reactions like, "I'm not crazy." To minimize the chances of offending the patient, the clinician should first explain the purpose of the inquiry and then ask initial broad questions. If the patient's responses are positive, then the clinician should follow up with more specific questions. The following is an example of the recommended strategy for screening for psychosis in mood disorders:

> *"When depression is really bad, some patients have unusual experiences. It may seem like their minds are playing tricks on them. Have you ever had any experiences like that?" or simply, "Have you ever had experiences that are hard to explain to others or are difficult to believe?"*

If the patient is uncertain or responds affirmatively, then the clinician should follow up with more direct, specific questions:

> *Have you ever heard sounds or voices that other people don't seem to hear?*
>
> *Do you ever feel paranoid?*

When the patient has had auditory hallucinations, it is important to inquire about their content. If a single voice does nothing more than occasionally call the patient's name, it is not a sign of psychosis and may be entirely normal. Multiple voices commenting on the patient's thoughts or behavior and conversing with each other is almost pathognomonic for schizophrenia. If the patient has experienced voices giving instructions or commands, then it is imperative to ask about commands to harm himself or others.

Assessing a Patient with Active Psychosis

Many patients with chronic schizophrenia have persistent hallucinations and delusions at their baseline despite treatment. Evaluating for change in their psychotic symptoms is more useful to evaluate for possible nonadherence or relapse than just eliciting specific symptoms. Most patients with schizophrenia have been coping with their psychotic experiences for many years and will share their coping strategies with health care providers if the patient trusts his or her provider. For someone with chronic paranoia, building trust is difficult; this may explain, in part, why many people with psychotic disorders do not keep regular medical appointments.

The great majority of psychotic patients are not violent, but there are important safety considerations in the assessment of an agitated psychotic patient, both for the safety of the interviewer and the safety of the patient. Whenever possible, such patients' evaluations should be relocated to an emergency department. A nonconfrontational approach that avoids escalating the patient's agitation is best. The following are some basic safety principles:

- Leave a clear exit to the door. Do not let the patient sit where he or she could impede your exit.
- Leave plenty of "personal space" for the patient. Do not crowd or inadvertently touch the patient. With his or her distorted internal reality, the patient could easily misinterpret these actions. Ask permission before beginning any physical examination.
- Use an even, clear voice that is easy to understand, and ask questions in short sentences. The patient may have difficulty following your conversation because of competing auditory hallucinations.

With these basic ideas in mind, ask direct questions about the reason for the visit and focus on the answers given. If the responses are organized and coherent, then proceed to more direct questions about any other symptoms. However, if the patient becomes more agitated and more disorganized, the clinician should consider terminating the interview and arranging for the patient to be taken to the nearest emergency department.

Treatment

Treatments for secondary psychotic symptoms (e.g., those that are substance-induced or due to a general medical condition) focus on finding the offending agent or disease and then addressing that. Stopping the medication that is causing the psychosis, correcting the hyponatremia, treating the seizure disorder, or managing benzodiazepine withdrawal are all in the realm of "treatments" for secondary psychoses. Delirium and dementia are discussed in Chapter 13, and substance-induced disorders are discussed in Chapter 12. Affective psychoses (i.e., psychosis associated with a mood disorder) are treated initially with an antipsychotic, typically in a hospital setting by a psychiatrist, and combined with either an antidepressant or mood stabilizers (i.e., for mania or bipolar depression with psychosis). (For more information about bipolar I, see Chapter 6.)

Schizophrenia

Schizophrenia is the most common of the disorders primarily presenting with psychotic symptoms and affects approximately 1% of the world's population. If related disorders are included (e.g., schizoaffective [0.7%] and delusional disorders [0.7%]), then the percentage is even greater. Given that schizophrenia starts in young adulthood and requires lifelong treatment, often with many hospitalizations, the economic burden is extreme. In 1990 the direct cost of care for schizophrenia in the United States was $33 billion, which exceeded all cancer treatment combined.

Schizophrenia affects men and women equally. On average, men have an earlier onset of symptoms (in their early 20s). Women present in their late 20s and are more likely to have affective symptoms. Prior to the onset of psychotic symptoms, there is usually a characteristic prodrome of decay in social functioning with eccentric ideas and behavior and social withdrawal, but this is often only recognized retrospectively (see Box 11-4). Patients with chronic schizophrenia have great difficulty functioning in society, and many (but not all) are unable to establish a stable domicile let alone maintain employment. There is a higher prevalence of schizophrenia in urban areas, probably accounted for by patients with schizophrenia who drift to the cities, where there are more psychiatric and social services available.

Box 11-4 Criteria for Schizophrenia

Two of the following for at least 1 month:

- Delusions
- Hallucinations
- Disorganized speech
- Grossly disorganized behavior
- Negative symptoms
- Significant impairment in functioning

Symptom complex and dysfunction that lasts for at least 6 months

The symptoms of schizophrenia are described as falling into 3 groups: positive symptoms, negative symptoms, and disorganized behavior. Positive symptoms include hallucinations and delusions. Negative (also called deficit) symptoms include restricted emotional expression, poverty of thought, lack of motivation, and lack of basic social skills, all of which often result in social isolation (see Table 11-1). Some patients with schizophrenia

Table 11-1 Positive and Negative Symptoms of Schizophrenia

Positive Symptoms	Negative Symptoms
Hallucinations	Flat, restricted affect
Delusions	Amotivation
Bizarre behavior	Poverty of thought
	Lack of basic social skills

present with primarily disorganized or bizarre behavior that is typically the product of their positive symptoms.

Course of Schizophrenia

Schizophrenia, which usually begins in early adulthood, can be divided into 3 phases: prodromal, acute, and residual. Frequently (but not always), there is a prodromal period lasting months to years with a crescendo of symptoms, beginning with eccentric ideas and behavior, progressing to deterioration in social functioning, social withdrawal, and eventually overt psychotic symptoms. The acute phase typically begins with an acute decompensation, including rapid increase in psychotic symptoms and decrease in ability to function, which is often precipitated by a stressful life event or substance abuse. Though the course is variable, the first 5 to 10 years is often a series of episodic exacerbations of positive symptoms and bizarre behavior, with further deterioration in functioning. Symptoms may resolve between exacerbations or simply diminish. Adherence to treatment is critical and linked to more favorable outcomes but is also very difficult to achieve. As the course of schizophrenia progresses, a plateauing of symptoms and relative stability is followed by a late or residual phase in which positive symptoms often diminish in intensity and some social functioning may be restored.

Schizophrenia and Comorbid Medical Disorders

The mortality rate in persons with schizophrenia is significantly higher than that of the general population. Suicide accounts for some of the excess mortality but not all. Infrequent preventive health care, combined with high rates of smoking and substance abuse, adds to their likelihood of dying earlier in life from a comorbid medical disease. When persons with schizophrenia are treated in mental health or primary care settings, they should be carefully screened for comorbid medical illnesses. Patients with schizophrenia have elevated rates of diabetes, hypertension, coronary artery disease, chronic obstructive pulmonary disease (COPD), and lung cancer, which may have been undetected or undertreated because of the patient's impairments in perception, communication, organization, and behavior.

Treatment of Schizophrenia

The ideal treatment of schizophrenia is the long-term combination of pharmacotherapy and psychosocial interventions involving family and community. Pharmacotherapy (i.e., neuroleptics; see Table 11-2) is essential and given for 4 reasons:

- To manage acute psychotic-symptom exacerbations
- To induce remission of symptoms
- To maintain remission
- To prevent relapse of psychotic symptoms

Table 11-2 Antipsychotics: Dosage

Agent	Starting Dose (mg)	Dose Range (mg)
Typical High Potency		
Haloperidol (Haldol)	0.5-5	5-15
Thiothixene (Navane)	2-5	10-30
Atypical		
Clozapine (Clozaril)	12.5 twice a day	25-300 three times a day
Risperidone (Risperdal)	0.5-1.0	0.5-4
Olanzapine (Zyprexa)	2.5-5.0	5.0-10
Quetiapine (Seroquel)	25	25-200
Ziprasidone (Geodon)	10-20	20-40
Aripiprazole (Abilify)	2.5-5.0	5-15

Adherence to medication is far more likely when accompanied by case management and integrated psychosocial treatment. Adherence is particularly difficult to achieve in schizophrenia because patients lack insight and even awareness that they are ill. There is some evidence that early pharmacologic treatment for schizophrenia and adherence with drug treatment improves the prognosis. Our discussion of treatment will focus on medications and particularly their potential adverse medical effects.

Antipsychotics and Neuroleptics

In 1952, the introduction of chlorpromazine (Thorazine) radically changed the treatment of schizophrenia. Until then, there were virtually no effective drugs for schizophrenia. Chlorpromazine ushered in the modern era of pharmacological management for schizophrenia and in large measure was what made deinstitutionalization possible, that is, shifting schizophrenics from chronic hospitalization in large institutions to the community.

Typical Antipsychotics: Low Potency

Chlorpromazine represents a group of antipsychotic agents referred to as typical, low-potency neuroleptics. They are "typical" in that they are thought to primarily work by blocking dopamine receptors in the brain; they are "low potency" in that high doses are required to achieve antipsychotic effects. These agents have anticholinergic, anti-alpha-adrenergic, and quinidine-like effects and subsequently are more likely to cause sedation, orthostasis, and cardiac side effects than typical, high-potency neuroleptics. Because they block dopamine, they also cause movement disorders, referred to as extrapyramidal side effects (EPS), but to a lesser degree than the high-potency agents (movement disorders are discussed further in this chapter). The reversible movement disorders include dystonia, akathisia, and Parkinsonism. The late-onset (tardive), often irreversible movement disorders include tardive dyskinesia (i.e., spontaneous abnormal movements), tardive dystonia, and tardive akathisia. The blockade of dopamine also releases the negative feedback of prolactin, and consequently prolactin levels rise, thereby contributing to sexual dysfunction and occasionally causing galactorrehea. Given these and other side effects, it is not hard to imagine why compliance is an issue. However, these agents were the backbone of treatment of psychotic disorders into the 1970s and are still used today, though less frequently.

Typical Antipsychotics: High Potency

In 1958, haloperidal (Haldol) was introduced. Like low-potency neuroleptics, haloperidol and the subsequent other high-potency neuroleptics also typically block dopamine receptors in the brain. However, high-potency neuroleptics work at much lower doses than their predecessors. High-potency neuroleptics have fewer anticholinergic, antiadrenergic, and cardiovascular side effects but increase the likelihood of movement disorders because of greater dopamine blockade. The risk of tardive movement disorders, particularly tardive dyskinesia (TD), presented a conundrum in the treatment of schizophrenia. All typical neuroleptics can cause irreversible tardive dyskinesia at rates of 25% to 40% of chronically treated patients but there were no effective alternatives for treating such a common and debilitating disorder.

Atypical or Novel Neuroleptics

Clozapine (Clozaril), introduced in the United States in 1989, was the first of a new generation of antipsychotic agents. Prior to clozapine, it was generally believed that psychosis was caused by excessive levels of dopamine in the brain and that the efficacy of typical neuroleptics was derived from their blockade of dopamine receptors (the dopamine hypothesis of schizophrenia). However, clozapine only weakly blocks D2 receptors. Clozapine blocked many other receptors but particularly serotonin receptors. Hence, these new neuroleptics have been referred to as "atypical" antipsychotics because their antipsychotic efficacy does not correlate with their ability to block dopamine receptors.

Clozapine turned out to have a potentially fatal side effect: it causes agranulocytosis in 1% of patients. Originally introduced in Europe in 1975, it was removed from the market until research demonstrated that clozapine was effective in some cases of schizophrenia unresponsive to other neuroleptics and that agranulocytosis could be prevented by checking the white blood cell count every week and discontinuing clozapine at the first sign of a dropping leukocyte count.

Though clozapine has other significant side effects in addition to agranulocytosis—including seizures, diabetes, weight gain, and cardiac side effects (e.g., orthostasis, tachycardia, rare fatal cardiomyopathy)—it does *not* appear to cause movement disorders. In fact, in some cases clozapine has improved patients' tardive movement symptoms. Patients treated with clozapine initially require weekly monitoring of the white blood cell count and frequent follow-ups to monitor for other side effects.

> **Box 11-5 Possible Major Side Effects of Antipsychotic Medications**
>
> ---
>
> Movement disorders
> Hypotension
> QTc prolongation
> Obesity
> Diabetes
> Hyperlipidemia
> Agranulocytosis
> Seizures
> Temperature dysregulation
> Hyperprolactinemia

Clozapine's success in treatment-resistant schizophenia and the absence of tardive dyskinesia led to the development and release of 5 atypical antipsychotic agents (listed in order of release in United States): risperidone (Risperdal), olanzapine (Zyprexa), quetiapine (Seroquel), ziprasidone (Geodon), and aripiprazole (Abilify). They all block both dopamine and serotonin but to varying degrees. General side effect patterns are reviewed in the next section (see Box 11-5).

Side Effects of Antipsychotic Medications
Movement Disorders Associated with Antipsychotics

Antipsychotics (especially the typical neuroleptics) cause reversible movement disorders, including dystonia, akathisia, and Parkinsonism, and irreversible movement disorders like tardive dyskinesia. Acute dystonia most often affects the muscles of the head and neck but can involve the entire body (opisthotonus). Acute dystonia may occur after a single parenteral dose of a neuroleptic or hours to days after an oral dose. Oral or intramuscular anticholinergic drugs like diphenhydramine (25-50 mg) or benztropine mesylate (Cogentin, 1-2 mg) will usually quickly relieve these symptoms. Akathisia can appear as restlessness, agitation, pacing, or feelings of electricity in the limbs and is very distressing for the patient. Akathisia may also occur soon after a single parenteral dose of a neuroleptic or days after an oral dose. Benzodiazepines and beta-blockers are usually most effective, but some patients also respond to anticholinergics. After weeks to months of treatment with antipsychotics, drug-induced Parkinsonism may occur, usually manifested in bradykinesia, cogwheel rigidity, and masked facies. This, too, usually responds to anticholinergic medication.

After years of treatment with neuroleptics, there is a risk of TD. Signs of TD include lip smacking, jutting tongue movements, grimacing, and excessive blinking (blepharospasm) as well as choreiform movements of the extremities. Rarely, TD involves the diaphragm and other muscles of respiration. There is no set course, and there is high variation from patient to patient. The risk factors for TD are influenced by the type of neuroleptic, the length of treatment, dosage, advanced age, and prior EPS. As already mentioned, typical antipsychotics, sometimes referred to as first-generation antipsychotics, carry a greater risk of TD than the newer atypical (second-generation) antipsychotics. It is estimated that typical antipsychotics carry approximately a 5% per year risk for TD (4,5). The risk may be as much as 3 to 5 times greater in patients older than 40 years (6). Kane, Chacos, and Woerner found that the risk of TD for 1, 2, and 3 years of typical antipsychotic exposure in neuroleptic-naive patients over 55 years was 25%, 34%, and 53%, respectively (4,5,6). Atypical antipsychotics carry a significantly decreased risk for TD, but how low the risk is remains unclear. The best current estimate is that the risk is about 1% per year. If TD is identified early, it may remit with cessation of the neuroleptic (usually requiring its replacement with clozapine). It should also be noted that not all dyskinesias encountered in patients treated with antipsychotics represent TD. Spontaneous dyskinesias occur in the elderly ("senile dykinesia") as part of other neurological disorders (e.g., Huntington disease, Sydenham chorea), as other side effects of other drugs (e.g., L-dopa), and possibly as a late consequence of schizophrenia itself.

The Abnormal Involuntary Movement Scale (AIMS) is used by many clinicians to follow any patient receiving an antipsychotic agent. It guides systematic assessment and scoring of abnormal movements and associated distress. Early detection of EPS permits intervention to provide relief, and early detection of TD may catch it while it is still reversible.

It is important to remember that antiemetic agents like prochlorperazine (Compazine) and promethazine (Phenergan) are low-potency phenothiazines like chlorpromazine and therefore can cause all of the same movement disorders caused by neuroleptics, including TD. This is also true of metoclopramide (Reglan), which blocks dopamine receptors, too.

Neuroleptic Malignant Syndrome

Neuroleptic malignant syndrome (NMS) is a rare but potentially fatal side effect of antipsychotics. NMS is characterized by elevated temperature (99°F-109°F), marked muscle rigidity, autonomic instability, altered mental status, markedly elevated creatine phosphokinase (CPK), and myoglobinuria. Treatment includes supportive measures (e.g., rapid cooling, hydration, muscle relaxants), immediate cessation of the neuroleptic, and avoidance of other dopamine-blocking drugs like antiemetics. While dantrolene and bromocriptine have been recommended by some, there is no clear evidence that they are superior to nonspecific supportive measures. ECT is effective in severe cases. Renal failure and respiratory failure can occur as a consequence of rhabdomyolysis or hyperthermia. The diagnosis can be difficult because the signs of NMS are nonspecific and the differential diagnosis is broad, including severe catatonia, heat stroke, and a variety of other febrile illnesses. NMS usually resolves 10 to 15 days after neuroleptic cessation (a month if the neuroleptic was a depot injection). NMS is not an absolute contraindication to reinstating an antipsychotic; generally an atypical antipsychotic is reinstituted at the lowest possible dose. Though all antipsychotics can cause NMS, it appears that typical, high-potency antipsychotics may carry the highest risk and atypical anti-psychotics carry the lowest risk (7).

Cardiovascular Side Effects

The most common cardiovascular side effect of antipsychotics is hypotension, which is common with low-potency, typical antipsychotics and clozapine. A potential quinidine-like effect of many antipsychotics is prolongation of the QTc interval, which may lead to the potentially fatal arrhythmia called torsades de pointes. Those at particular risk include patients with a pre-existing familial long QT syndrome and those who develop undue QTc prolongation during treatment with other QTc-prolonging drugs such as TCAs. A pretreatment electrocardiogram is indicated for patients who have a personal or family history of sudden death or syncope or a personal history of heart disease, hypokalemia, hypomagnesemia, or other significant cardiac risk factors. Among antipsychotics, pimozide, thioridazine, droperidol, and ziprasidone carry the highest risk for prolonging the QTc interval. Although even haloperidol has caused QTc prolongation, especially when parenterally administered at a high dose, it is generally accepted to be minimally cardiotoxic.

Both relative and absolute increases in the risk of sudden death were observed in patients taking moderate doses of typical antipsychotics (8). Increasing the dosage of the antipsychotic and concurrent cardiovascular disease significantly increase the risk of cardiac sudden death. However, the increase may not be attributable to all neuroleptics because schizophrenics have high rates of smoking, poor health care, obesity, and diabetes—all significant factors impacting cardiac disease.

Clozapine is the only antipsychotic known to cause potentially fatal myocarditis, often resulting in a dilated cardiomyopathy. Estimated rates range from 1 in 500 to 1 in 10,000. Eighty-five percent of the cases develop during the first 2 months of therapy.

Weight Gain and Obesity

Obesity is a growing concern in the United States and other developed countries. Because of sedentary lifestyle and poor dietary habits, chronically psychotic patients are at an increased risk for obesity. While most antipsychotics can cause weight gain, the problem has received much more attention since the advent of the atypical antipsychotics. The risk and degree of weight gain varies among both typical and atypical antipsychotics. Low-potency, typical antipsychotics are much more likely to cause weight gain than high-potency ones. While precise data on relative risk among the atypicals are not available, it is clear that clozapine and olanzapine carry the greatest liability for weight gain, followed by quetiapine and risperidone. Aripiprazole and ziprasidone appear to be weight neutral. Most of the weight gain occurs relatively early (i.e., the first 10 weeks) and then plateaus, but the gains can be considerable in a minority of patients (e.g., 20-25 kg). Weight gain appears to result both from an increase in appetite and changes in metabolism.

The primary treatment approach to this potential weight gain is behavioral. Patients should be informed that appetite will potentially increase during initial therapy, and they should be educated regarding dietary and activity steps that can help prevent weight gain.

Diabetes and Hyperlipidemia

Closely related to weight gain are the concerns of diabetes and hyperlipidemia. Some of the atypical antipsychotics significantly increase risk for diabetes and hyperlipidemia, and some of this risk is independent of weight gain. It should also be noted that for unknown reasons there is an increased risk for diabetes in schizophrenia and bipolar disorder irrespective of treatment. Clozapine clearly poses the greatest risk, followed in order by olanzapine, risperidone, and quetiapine. Aripiprazole and ziprasidone have not been shown to be associated with an increased incidence of hyperglycemia. In most cases of atypical antipsychotic-induced hyperglycemia, the risk of hyperglycemia is not dose related and typically occurs early in treatment (i.e., 10 days to 3 months) and reverts when the antipsychotic is stopped. Current recommendations include measurement of pretreatment fasting glucose and careful monitoring in patients at increased risk for type II diabetes as well as those who already have diabetes.

Hyperlipidemia (hypercholesterolemia and elevated triglycerides) has been associated most often with clozapine and olanzapine, less often with quetiapine and risperidone, and not with ziprasidone or aripiprazole. Low-potency, typical antipsychotics, but not high-potency ones, may also cause hyperlipidemia.

Other Significant Side Effects

Hematologic side effects of antipsychotics have included agranulocytosis, aplastic anemia, neutropenia, eosinophilia, and thrombocytopenia. Such effects are rare with antipsychotics other than clozapine. Clozapine-associated agranulocytosis occurs in 1% to 2% of patients, with the highest risk in the first 6 months, but it is impossible to predict if and when it will occur.

All antipsychotics lower seizure thresholds. The risk is lowest for high-potency, typical antipsychotics and risperidone (0.5%) and is intermediate with olanzapine, quetiapine, and low-potency, typical antipsychotics. The highest risk is with clozapine (1%-2%, and perhaps as high as 5% at high doses).

All antipsychotics may interfere with temperature regulation. One form of this is NMS, which was previously discussed. All antipsychotics can also cause heat stroke, a major risk in poorly ventilated housing or prolonged exposure in hot climates.

Hyperprolactinemia is most common with high-potency, typical antipsychotics and risperidone and can result in amenorrhea or irregular menses, galactorrhea, gynecomastia, sexual dysfunction, and osteoporosis.

Informed Consent and Documentation

When considering any therapy, clinicians must balance the risks of treatment vs the benefits. The greater the risk of treatment, the greater the duty to warn, monitor, and seek alternative approaches. The occurrence of neuroleptic-induced tardive dyskinesia has prompted many psychiatrists to take added care when obtaining and documenting informed consent prior to prescribing an antipsychotic. General clinicians should follow similar practices guided by some common sense. First, short-term usage of low-dose antipsychotics (both typical and atypical, other than clozapine) carries a relatively low risk of irreversible or otherwise serious side effects. However, if an antipsychotic is prescribed for continuous indefinite usage, then documented, informed consent is recommended (meaning documenting that the patient understands the reasons for taking the drug, its risks, and its benefits). This is often not possible when a patient is acutely psychotic and must be postponed until there has been sufficient recovery. When prescribing responsibility for antipsychotic medication is transferred to a primary care clinician from a psychiatrist, one should not presume that that the psychiatrist documented the patient's consent previously; even if he or she did, the patient may have no recall of it.

KEY POINTS

- Psychosis in the primary care setting is more likely to be caused by a nonpsychotic disorder (e.g., psychotic depression, mania with psychosis) than by a psychotic disorder (e.g., schizophrenia).
- Hallucinations can occur across all 5 senses.
- Visual hallucinations are more common in organic psychoses but also occur in psychiatrically based psychoses.
- Organic psychoses are most likely when tactile, gustatory, and olfactory hallucinations are present.
- In schizophrenia, positive symptoms include hallucinations and delusions. Negative symptoms include emotional blunting, poverty of thought and speech, and avolitional or amotivational behavior.
- "Typical" neuroleptics refer to first-generation antipsychotics, which produce strong dopamine blockade.
- "Atypical" neuroleptics refer to newer antipsychotics, which have diverse effects on serotonin and dopamine receptors.

- Typical antipsychotics are associated with movement disorders, both short-term and long-term.
- Atypical antipsychotics are much less likely to cause movement disorders but can cause other serious side effects including weight gain, diabetes, and hyperlipidemia.
- Informed consent should be documented in the medical record of patients prescribed an antipsychotic for an extended period.

REFERENCES

1. Webster R, Holroyd S. Prevalence of psychotic symptoms in delirium. *Psychosomatics*. 2000;41:519-523.
2. Masand PS, Christopher E, Clary GL, et al. Mania, catatonia, and psychosis in the medically ill. In: Levenson JL, ed. *The American Psychiatric Publishing Textbook of Psychosomatic Medicine*. Washington, DC: American Psychiatric Publishing, Inc; 2005:235-250.
3. Goldberg JF, Harrow M, Whiteside JE. Risk for bipolar illness in patients initially hospitalized for unipolar depression. *Am J Psychiatry*. 2001;158:1265-1270.
4. Kane JM, Honigfeld G, Singer J, et al. Clozapine for the treatment-resistant schizophrenic: a double-blind comparison versus chlorpromazine/benztropine. *Arch Gen Psychiatry*. 1998;45:789.
5. Chakos MH, Alvir JM, Woerner MG, et al. Incidence and correlates of tardive dyskinesia in first episode of schizophrenia. *Arch of Gen Psych*. 1996;53:313-319.
6. Woerner MG, Alvir JM, Saltz BL, et al. Prospective study of tardive dyskinesia in the elderly: rates and risk factors. *Am J Psychiatry*. 1998;155:1521-1528.
7. Pelonero AL, Levinson JL, Pandurangi AK. Neuroleptic malignant syndrome: a review. *Psychiatric Services*. 1998;49:1163.
8. Ray WA, Meredith S, Thapa PB, et al. Antipsychotics and the risk of sudden cardiac death. *Arch Gen Psychiatry*. 2001;58:1161-1167.

KEY REFERENCES

Aleman A, Agrawal N, Morgan KD, et al. Insight in psychosis and neuropsychological function: meta-analysis. *Br J Psychiatry*. 2006;189:204-212.

Fenton WS. Prevalence of spontaneous dyskinesia in schizophrenia. *J Clin Psychiatry*. 2000;61(4):10-14.

Glassman AH, Bigger JT Jr. Antipsychotic drugs: prolonged QTc interval, torsade de pointes, and sudden death. *Am J Psychiatry*. 2001;158:1774-1782.

Joy CB, Adams CE, Lawrie SM. Haloperidol versus placebo for schizophrenia. *Cochrane Database Syst Rev*. 2006;(4):CD003082.

Lieberman JA, Stroup TS, McEvoy JP, et al. Clinical Antipsychotic Trials of Intervention Effectiveness (CATIE) Investigators. Effectiveness of antipsychotic drugs in patients with chronic schizophrenia. *N Engl J Med*. 2005;353(12):1209-1223.

Perala J, Suvisaari J, Saarni SI, et al. Lifetime prevalence of psychotic and bipolar I disorders in a general population. *Arch Gen Psychiatry*. 2007;64(1):19-28.

Ramaswamy K, Masand PS, Nasrallah HA. Do certain atypical antipsychotics increase the risk of diabetes? A critical review of 17 pharmacoepidemiologic studies. *Ann Clin Psychiatry*. 2006;18(3):183-194.

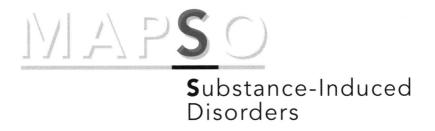

Substance-Induced Disorders

■ Chapter 12 **Substance Use and Psychiatric Disorders**

S

■ Substance-Induced Disorders ▬▬▬▬▬▬▬▬▬▬▬▬▬▬▬▬▬▬▬

Substance Use and Psychiatric Disorders

■ Substance Use in Patients with Psychiatric Disorders and the Role of the General Clinician

Substance-related problems of psychiatric relevance include substance abuse (here used broadly to include DSM-IV abuse and dependence), intoxication syndromes, withdrawal syndromes, and substance-induced psychiatric disorders. The latter includes not only alcohol and classic substances of abuse but also prescribed medications like interferons and corticosteroids. Consistent with the purposes of this book, we have primarily focused on issues relevant to general clinicians in caring for patients with psychiatric disorders. The reader is referred to other sources for detailed reviews of the diagnosis and management of primary substance-related disorders.

In this chapter, we first review the basic terminology of addiction, abuse, and dependence. Next we look at how the effects and side effects of some commonly used medications (e.g., corticosteroids and interferons) can cause psychiatric disorders. Finally we examine the interactions between comorbid substance use and psychiatric disorders with particular focus on caffeine use, nicotine dependence and depression, and moderate alcohol use in patients with psychiatric disorders.

S

■ Essential Concepts and Terms

Abuse, Dependence, and Addiction

Precision in definitions and terminology is important in guiding diagnosis and treatment. Casual misuse of terms by any clinician can result in false-positive and false-negative diagnoses of substance-related disorders as well as stigmatization of patients. Abuse, tolerance, withdrawal, dependence, and addiction may occur not only with alcohol and illegal substances but also with a variety of prescription and nonprescription medications.

Substance Abuse

According to the DSM-IV, substance abuse is defined as a maladaptive pattern of substance use leading to clinically significant impairment or distress and is manifested by 1 or more of the following criteria occurring in a 12-month period:

1. Recurrent substance use resulting in failure to fulfill major obligations at work, school, or home
2. Recurrent substance use in situations that could be physically hazardous (e.g., driving or operating machinery)
3. Recurrent substance-related legal problems
4. Continued substance use despite having persistent, recurrent social or interpersonal problems caused or exacerbated by the substance

Tolerance

Tolerance is the need for an ever-increasing amount of a substance to achieve the desired effect or a markedly diminished effect with continued use of the substance of the same quantity.

Withdrawal

Withdrawal is defined as the generally unpleasant symptoms that are experienced when blood or tissue concentrations of the substance decline.

Please note that tolerance and withdrawal, the 2 hallmarks of dependence, can occur when substances are abused as well as when the same substances are used appropriately. All patients receiving chronic daily opioid therapy develop tolerance and will experience withdrawal symptoms if the drug is abruptly stopped, but most have simple *physiologic* dependence and do not misuse or abuse opioids or develop the *disorder* of dependence as defined next.

Substance Dependence

Substance dependence is defined by the DSM-IV as a maladaptive pattern of substance use leading to clinically significant impairment as manifested by 3 or more of the following occurring at any time in the same 12-month period:

1. Tolerance is experienced.
2. Withdrawal is experienced.
3. The substance is often taken in larger amounts or over a longer period than intended.
4. There is a persistent desire or there are unsuccessful efforts to cut down or control use of the substance.
5. A great deal of time is spent in activities necessary to obtain the substance.
6. An important social occupation or recreational activities are given up or reduced because of the substance.
7. The substance is used despite knowledge of its negative consequences.

Addiction

In the past, addiction was a term used exclusively for substance addiction, but now the concept has been expanded to behavioral addictions such as compulsive gambling, shopping, sexual activity, eating, and viewing Internet pornography. This chapter does not address behavioral addictions. Though an official DSM-IV definition of addiction does not exist at this time, addiction is the compulsive physiological and psychological need for a habit-forming substance. Those who are addicted use a substance on a regular basis that produces pleasure or provides escape from internal discomfort. However, the individual feels powerless to stop use of the substance, and the substance use is continued despite significant negative consequences in the individual's life. Therefore, all forms of addiction share common symptoms including craving, loss of control, and impairment.

Pseudo-addiction

Pseudo-addiction refers to the situation in which a patient increases the dose of a prescribed medication to attempt to relieve symptoms that are not being adequately relieved by the prescribed dose. This is not uncommon with opioid pain medications that are given at inadequate doses or frequency. Therefore, to continue to function and to compensate for the increased pain, the patient increases his or her dose of pain medication and then asks for earlier refill or a new prescription, exhibiting "drug-seeking behavior" reminiscent of someone with true substance addiction.

Psychiatric Symptoms Caused by Non-abused Medications

Many substances can induce neuropsychiatric symptoms by intoxication (as a side effect or a result of toxicity), withdrawal (due to abrupt cessation), or long-term effects. The phenomena of substance-induced disorders mimicking psychiatric disorders have been noted in previous chapters describing mood, anxiety, and psychotic disorders. Chronic use of most abused substances—particularly alcohol, sedative-hypnotics, cocaine, and amphetamines—frequently produces depressive symptoms. But it is also common for depressed patients to seek escape from their depression through substance abuse. A 48-year-old man presents with gastritis, and his clinician determines that the patient has been drinking heavily on a daily basis for years and appears to be quite depressed. How does one determine whether his depression is due to his drinking or his drinking is due to his depression? While a careful history, including information from his wife, may shed light on the answer, it is usually the case that the only way to be certain is to observe the patient after a period of abstinence. If his mood improves, then he likely has a depression caused, or least aggravated, by alcohol.

Gross intoxication and full-blown withdrawal syndromes are familiar to most clinicians, but subtler presentations can be easily mistaken for primary psychiatric disorders. Chronic marijuana use may cause symptoms that mimic attention deficit disorder or depression. Acute or chronic generalized anxiety and panic attacks may be caused by cocaine or amphetamines or by withdrawal from alcohol or sedative-hypnotics.

In addition to substances of abuse, patients in primary care settings are frequently taking many medications that alone or in combination may cause psychiatric symptoms. We will illustrate this by focusing on caffeine, interferons, and corticosteroids.

Interferon-Induced Psychiatric Symptoms

Interferons are frequently used in the treatment of hepatitis C infections and malignancies including malignant melanoma. These treatments, particularly for hepatitis C, may be life-saving. However, some patients develop interferon-induced depression. In fact, the most common reason for discontinuation of interferon treatment for hepatitis C is interferon-induced depression. Further, many of the patients with chronic hepatitis C have a premorbid history of (or vulnerability to) psychiatric illness, particularly major depression and substance abuse. Several well-designed prospective studies (1,2) have shown a causal association between interferon use and mood disorders (mainly major depression). Mood symptoms like irritability, depression, and fatigue occur in 33% to 50% of patients, while interferon-induced major depression has been reported in up to one third of patients. Anxiety-like symptoms occur in about 20% of patients. Interferon-induced depression can be severe, and there have been many case reports of suicide and suicide attempts during interferon treatment of hepatitis C, multiple sclerosis, and other diseases.

A 2001 randomized, controlled prevention trial demonstrated that pretreatment with the SSRI antidepressant paroxetine in patients with malignant melanoma who were receiving interferon significantly reduced the incidence of depression. Specifically, major depression developed in only 11% of the paroxetine group and in 45% of the placebo group. Of most importance, severe depression led to the discontinuation of interferons in only 5% of the paroxetine group, whereas 35% of the placebo group stopped interferon treatment because of severe depression (3).

Some experts have subsequently advocated that all patients receiving interferons treatment should be prophylactically treated with an antidepressant—even those with no prior depression. Currently, however, this has not been proven effective in chronic hepatitis C and does not constitute standard practice. It is generally accepted that patients with a prior history of depression should have antidepressant therapy initiated prior to starting interferons.

The clinician should remember the following guidelines when dealing with patients receiving interferon treatment:

- Prior to treatment with interferons, screen for current and prior psychiatric illness, especially major mood disorders.
- If a strong history of major mood disorders exists, then begin pretreatment with an antidepressant. SSRIs are the most commonly used antidepressants in patients with hepatitis C.
- If major mood symptoms appear, suicide risk should be assessed and treatment with an antidepressant should be immediately initiated and titrated up to a therapeutic dose.
- Patients with a prior history of depression should have antidepressant therapy initiated prior to starting interferon treatment.

Corticosteroid-Induced Psychiatric Symptoms

Approximately 10 million *new* prescriptions are written for oral cortico-steroids each year in the United States, which does not include standing prescriptions, long-term use, or intravenous steroids used in hospitals. In many patients, corticosteroids enhance a feeling of well-being, which can even lead to steroid overuse and, rarely, dependence. Shortly after the introduction of corticosteroid therapy, numerous case reports and case series were published describing many psychiatric symptoms, including depressed mood; unstable mood swings; mania and hypomanic symptoms (e.g., increased energy, decreased sleep, agitation, rapid speech, and, in severe cases, grandiosity and flight of ideas); psychosis with hallucinations; delusional beliefs and disorganized thoughts; and even suicidal ideation.

All of these psychiatric symptoms associated with corticosteroid use have collectively been referred to as "steroid psychosis." This terminology is misleading because most patients experiencing psychiatric adverse effects of corticosteroids (e.g., mood symptoms of depression, irritability, and elation are the most common) are not psychotic (i.e., they do not expe-rience hallucinations or delusions).

A recent review of 2 large meta-analyses examining psychiatric symp-toms in patients taking corticosteroids reported rates of moderate and severe "reactions" (including psychosis) as 23% and 6%, respectively (4). The most common symptoms during short courses of corticosteroids were euphoria and hypomania, and in chronic treatment the most common were depressive symptoms. The likelihood of adverse reactions was directly related to dosage (i.e., the higher the dose, the more likely the adverse reactions). Prospective studies have supported the causal association between corticosteroids and psychiatric symptoms, though the occurrence of full-criteria psychiatric disorders is relatively infrequent when compared to 1 or 2 isolated psychiatric (e.g., mood) symptoms.

With the high prevalence of steroid-induced mood symptoms, it is important for the clinician to actively monitor patients receiving corticos-teroids for their occurrence, particularly euphoria and hypomania. The evi-dence guiding treatment of corticosteroid-induced psychiatric symptoms is sparse and anecdotal. If significant mood symptoms do occur, then reduc-ing the dose or stopping the corticosteroid will usually resolve the symp-toms. If steroid treatment must be sustained, manic symptoms have usually been treated with mood stabilizers (e.g., lithium, valproic acid, or carba-mazepine), while antipsychotics, with their more rapid onset of action, have been used for acute and more severe reactions (e.g., psychosis, extreme mania, or delirium). Antidepressants for corticosteroid-induced depression should be used cautiously because they may sometimes induce a switch to mania. (See Chapter 6 for more on cycling and bipolar disor-ders.) Because of this, we recommend that the use of antidepressants be reserved for patients receiving long-term corticosteroids who cannot reduce their dose of corticosteroids. Antidepressants should not be used without a mood stabilizer in the treatment of corticosteroid-induced major depression in patients with a previous history of mania regardless of whether the mania was spontaneous or steroid-induced.

The following summarizes what is known regarding steroid-induced psychiatric symptoms:

■ In many patients, corticosteroids enhance one's feeling of well-being.
■ The higher the dose, the greater the likelihood of moderate or severe adverse reactions.
■ Psychiatric diagnoses that meet the full criteria for major depression or bipolar I disorder (with psychosis) are fairly rare and usually resolve with cessation or decrease of the corticosteroid dose.
■ Symptoms of mania and psychosis tend to come earlier in the course of treatment with corticosteroids.
■ Symptoms of depression tend to come later in the course of treatment with corticosteroids.
■ When corticosteroids cannot be stopped, psychotropic medication should be targeted to the particular psychiatric side effects.

Caffeine-Induced Psychiatric Symptoms

Caffeine is the most common psychoactive substance in the world, most often ingested through coffees, teas, "energy drinks," and sodas, but caffeine is also contained in many over-the-counter remedies for headache, fatigue, and weight loss, for example. When caffeine is consumed acutely, usually in excess of 250 mg (i.e., the amount in more than 2 to 3 cups of brewed coffee), symptoms of caffeine intoxication may occur (e.g., restlessness, nervousness, excitement, insomnia, flushed face, GI disturbances, psychomotor agitation, and rapid speech).

When caffeine is ingested chronically, a high degree of tolerance occurs. Cessation frequently provokes withdrawal symptoms. In some people, caffeine can induce addiction-like symptoms such as craving and organizing one's behavior toward its regular consumption. As with many other addictive substances, caffeine use may be continued chronically to avoid withdrawal symptoms.

Though the DSM-IV does not recognize caffeine dependence as a clinical entity, signs and symptoms of withdrawal from caffeine are well documented and include tachycardia, decreased motor activity, headache, fatigue, and lethargy. The incidence of withdrawal symptoms after caffeine deprivation in regular users of caffeine has been reported to be between 35% and 100%. In a population-based survey of caffeine users, over 40% reported experiencing 1 or more withdrawal symptoms; the study included users who had stopped or cut down caffeine use for at least 24 hours in the past year (5).

The following are our recommendations regarding caffeine use:

- Obtain a careful history of caffeine use with special attention to any changes in use during the time of the psychiatric symptoms.
- Avoid sudden cessation of caffeine, especially if initiating medications.
- If there is enough suspicion that caffeine may be causing or compounding symptoms, then request a 3-month trial of no caffeine to see if symptoms change during the trial.

The Interface Between Comorbid Substance Use and Psychiatric Disorders

Substance use and abuse are very common in most psychiatric disorders and can have a number of negative effects on symptoms and treatment. Substance abuse is one of the most common explanations for treatment failure yet is often unrecognized or ignored. Substance abuse results in poor adherence with treatment, poor sleep, disruption of social networks, medical complications, and other adverse effects.

Caffeine Use in Patients with Psychiatric Disorders

While quantification of caffeine use should be routinely included in the medical history of every patient, it becomes much more significant when the patient also has psychiatric symptoms. Every patient with anxiety or mood symptoms should be asked how much caffeine they are consuming. While not usually the sole cause of anxiety, caffeine is a frequent aggravator. Patients with chronic depression, insomnia, or fatigue often overuse caffeine to improve energy and overcome lethargy, but excessive caffeine depletes energy and disrupts sleep, in turn aggravating the original condition. Chronic overuse of caffeine resulting in irritability, labile mood, and overstimulation may be mistaken for hypomania.

Caffeine consumption should be considered when initiating many psychiatric medications. Activating agents like bupropion, SSRIs, and SNRIs have produced significant symptoms of anxiety and agitation when initiated in patients consuming significant amounts of caffeine. Conversely, the sudden cessation of all caffeinated beverages can induce withdrawal symptoms that can mimic or can exacerbate side effects of the drug being initiated. As with patients in whom caffeine is causing psychiatric symptoms, a 3-month trial of no caffeine should be considered when it is suspected that caffeine is aggravating psychiatric symptoms.

S

Nicotine Use in Patients with Depression

Most clinicians are familiar with nicotine dependence and the subsequent health risks. Smoking cessation and the modalities used to overcome nicotine addiction are part of most general medical curricula. (See Key References at the end of the chapter.)

Most clinicians, however, are not familiar with the increased incidence and prevalence of depression in people who smoke and the adverse effects of depression on the patient's ability to stop smoking. The odds that a smoker will be depressed are about 3 times the odds for a nonsmoker. If a smoker has a history of major depression, he or she is more likely to experience a recurrence of his or her depression after stopping smoking as compared with smokers who do not have a history of major depression. In one study, for smokers with no prior history of major depression, the 3-month incidence of a new major depression after smoking cessation was 2%; for those with a single prior episode of major depression the incidence of depression was 17%; and in individuals with recurrent major depression, the incidence of another episode was 30% (6).

The following are recommendations for clinicians working with patients who smoke and are considering cessation:

- First, assess if the patient currently has major depression. If so, treat the depression before proceeding with smoking cessation.
- Second, obtain a detailed past history for depression and other psychiatric disorders. Successful cessation is less likely for smokers with past depression, so nicotine replacement, bupropion, varenicline, or behavior therapy are more likely to be needed. No medication has been shown to be effective for smoking cessation without concomitant behavior change.
- Third, people who have experienced past depression are in need of closer monitoring for symptoms of depression during smoking cessation and should be educated to be on the watch for such symptoms.

Any antidepressant can be used to treat depression in smokers; one should not automatically choose bupropion. After remission is achieved for the depression, many patients will want to stop smoking. Adding bupropion or nicotine replacement to their medication regimen may be helpful but should be done with caution because of the increased likelihood of additive side effects. For smoking cessation, bupropion sustained release (SR) is frequently started at 150 mg daily and then increased to twice daily in 3 to 5 days. This is too much and too fast for a patient already on another antidepressant. To avoid unwanted side effects and reduce the chances of early failure of smoking cessation, start bupropion SR at a lower dose (i.e., 100 mg) once daily and titrate the dose up slowly, every 2 weeks if tolerated.

There is no published experience using the new smoking cessation aid varenicline in patients with depression.

Is There Appropriate Use of Alcohol in a Patient with a Psychiatric Disorder?

The following discussion assumes that the patient has no active or past history of substance abuse; if there is a history of abuse, then the recommendation is to abstain from all alcohol. The more common situation is a patient recovering from a psychiatric disorder who inquires about whether it is safe to drink while taking his or her psychiatric medication. There is not much information to guide the clinician in this situation.

Every package insert warns about alcohol use with any psychiatric drug. What frequently happens is there is either no discussion about alcohol use or a recommendation of total abstinence from all alcohol. Our recommendation is to engage the patient in a discussion about alcohol use and review what we do know about the risks and how to apply this information to his or her unique case.

The first concept is that the greater the number of medications and the more severe the disorder, then the greater the risk of any alcohol intake. Some medications should not be mixed with alcohol. Benzodiazepines are the most obvious example because they have potentially severe interactions with alcohol, ranging from increased sedation to respiratory depression. Multiple medications only compound the risk of a negative interaction with alcohol. Also, some psychiatric disorders (e.g., bipolar disorder) have such a high comorbid rate of substance abuse that alcohol should be avoided.

The second concept is to avoid all alcohol (and all psychoactive drugs) both before initiating treatment and while initiating medications. In circumstances in which it is not clear whether the patient's symptoms are substance-induced or a disorder, suggest an "experiment" of abstinence for all psychoactive substances (including alcohol) for a month and monitor for any change in symptoms. If a medication is initiated, then cessation of all alcohol is critical so that accurate assessments for medication effects and side effects is not confounded with effects from alcohol.

The third concept is understanding how and when some alcohol intake can occur for some patients with psychiatric disorders. Many psychiatric disorders require chronic treatment with medication whose aim is to achieve symptom-free remission. The most common example is recurrent major depression that is in maintenance-phase treatment with an antidepressant. Patients should be instructed that the antidepressant may magnify the effects of alcohol, and the alcohol may influence the effects of the antidepressant. Specifically, the patient's sensitivity to even small quantities of alcohol may be heightened. Also, side effects from antidepressants, including nausea and headache, may be increased. The last part of this discussion with the patient should include reference to a growing body of literature that notes that even moderate *regular* intake of alcohol is associated with poorer long-term outcomes for depression when compared to total abstinence. Most people, however, can take an *occasional* drink without ill effects. The following are our recommendations for clinicians:

■ Review alcohol consumption with the patient in terms of risk (e.g., relapse of psychiatric symptoms, potential heightened effects of alcohol, and interactions with psychotropic medications).
■ Instruct the patient not to consume alcohol daily.

- Have the patient limit alcohol consumption to no more than twice weekly.
- If or when alcohol is consumed, instruct the patient to limit consumption to 1 or 2 drinks and no more.
- Document in the patient's medical record your discussions regarding alcohol and prospectively monitor it with subsequent notations in the medical record.

Overall, less alcohol is better than more alcohol, and a healthy lifestyle that includes exercise and weight control is best.

■ Case-Finding Strategies

Case-finding strategies begin with the clinician first considering that all or some of the patient's presenting symptoms may be caused (i.e., "induced") or exacerbated by some ingested substance. The major offending agents include prescribed or over-the-counter medications, closely followed by substances associated with abuse and dependence (e.g., alcohol, nicotine, caffeine). The general clinician should routinely review *all* medications and be familiar with their psychiatric side effects. Reviewing *all* psychoactive substances with the patient is key. If regular ingestion (i.e., use) is occurring, then clearly delineating the quantity and frequency will help determine if the substance may have a causal or complicating role in the presenting symptoms. The following represent some general questions that may prove helpful:

Are you taking any over-the-counter medications, vitamins, or supplements?

Do you drink caffeinated drinks? Daily? What kind? How much? Have you changed (increased or stopped) your usage recently? What happens if you do not consume this?

When was your last drink of beer, wine, or any alcoholic beverage? How much did you have? What is the greatest amount you have consumed in one sitting in the last month? Have you recently changed the amount you consume?

Have you recently increased or decreased your smoking? Why? How did that affect you?

■ Treatment

Treatments for substance abuse and dependence are beyond the scope of this chapter. The reader is referred to the references at the end of the chapter for further information.

KEY POINTS

- Consider all psychoactive substances and not just substances of abuse.
- Addiction is the compulsive physiological and psychological need for a habit-forming substance.
- Dependence is substance abuse plus evidence of physiological dependence (e.g., tolerance, withdrawal).
- Abuse is continued substance use despite interference in functioning.
- Pseudo-addiction is an increase in the dose (i.e., use) of a prescribed medication by a patient to attempt to relieve symptoms that are not being adequately relieved by the prescribed dose.
- Corticosteroids are one of the most frequently used medications that can cause psychiatric symptoms.
- "Steroid psychosis" refers to all psychiatric symptoms associated with corticosteroid use.
- Interferons produce significant psychiatric symptoms that frequently lead to cessation of the interferon therapy.
- Treating depression before interferon therapy dramatically reduces the dropout rate from depression.
- Caffeine is the most frequently ingested psychoactive agent.
- Symptoms of caffeine withdrawal and intoxication frequently complicate treatment of psychiatric disorders.
- Depression has a significant negative impact on successful smoking cessation.
- Bupropion and nicotine replacement is efficacious but may cause significant side effects, especially when given concurrently with an antidepressant.
- Abstinence from alcohol is recommended when a patient has a past history of substance abuse, is taking multiple medications (e.g., benzodiazepines), has severe symptoms of the disorder, or is initiating treatment.
- Asymptomatic patients in maintenance-phase treatments may consume limited amounts of alcohol after discussion with the general clinician.

References

1   Asnis GM, De La Garza R II. Interferon-induced depression in chronic hepatitis C: a review of its prevalence, risk factors, biology, and treatment approaches. *J Clin Gastroenterol.* 2006;40:322-335.

2. Loftis JM, Hauser P. The phenomenology and treatment of interferon-induced depression. *J Affect Disord.* 2004;82:175-190

3. Musselman DL, Lawson DH, Gumnick JF, et al. Paroxetine for the prevention of depression induced by high-dose interferon alfa. *N Engl J Med.* 2001;344:961-966.

4. Warrington TP, Bostwick JM. Psychiatric adverse effects of corticosteroids. *Mayo Clin Proc.* 2006;81:1361-1367.

5. Dews PB, Curtis GL, Hanford KJ, et al. The frequency of caffeine withdrawal in a population-based survey and in a controlled, blinded pilot experiment. *J Clin Pharmacol.* 1999;39(12):1221-1232.

6. Covey LS, Glassman AH, Stetner F. Major depressive disorder following smoking cessation. *Am J Psychiatry.* 1997;154:263-265.

Key References

American Psychiatric Association. Practice guideline for the treatment of patients with substance use disorders: alcohol, cocaine, opioids. *Am J Psychiatry.* 1995;152:1-59.

American Psychiatric Association. Practice guideline for the treatment of patients with nicotine dependence. *Am J Psychiatry.* 1996;153:1-31.

Blondal T, Gudmundsson LJ, Olafsdottir I, et al. Nicotine nasal spray with nicotine patch for smoking cessation: randomised trial with six year follow up. *BMJ.* 1999;318:285-288.

Bradley KA, Boyd-Wickizer J, Powell SH, et al. Alcohol screening questionnaires in women: a critical review. *JAMA.* 1998;280:166-171.

Castaneda R, Sussman N, Westreich L, et al. A review of the effects of moderate alcohol intake on the treatment of anxiety and mood disorders. *J Clin Psychiatry.* 1996;57(5):207-212.

Franklin JE, Levenson JL, McCance-Katz EF. Substance-related disorders. In: Levenson JL, ed. *American Psychiatric Publishing Textbook of Psychosomatic Medicine.* Washington, DC: American Psychiatric Publishing, Inc; 2005:387-422.

Hughes JR, Oliveto AH, Bickel WK, et al. Caffeine self-administration and withdrawal: incidence, individual differences and interrelationships. *Drug Alcohol Depend.* 1993;32:239-246.

Hughes JR, Oliveto AH, Ligouri A, et al. Endorsement of DSM-IV dependence criteria among caffeine users. *Drug Alcohol Depend.* 1998;52(2):99-107.

Ko DT, Hebert PR, Coffey CS, et al. ß-blocker therapy and symptoms of depression, fatigue, and sexual dysfunction. *JAMA.* 2002;288:351-357.

Okuyemi KS, Nollen NL, Ahluwalia JS. Interventions to facilitate smoking cessation. *Am Fam Physician.* 2006;74(2):262-271.

Ried LD, McFarland BH, Johnson RE, et al. Beta-blockers and depression: the more the murkier? *The Annals of Pharmacotherapy.* 1998;32:699-708.

Srivastava P, Currie GP, Britton J. Smoking cessation. *BMJ.* 2006332(7553):1324-1326.

Wada K, Yamada N, Suzuki H, et al. Recurrent cases of corticosteroid-induced mood disorder: clinical characteristics and treatment. *J Clin Psychiatry.* 2000;61:261-267.

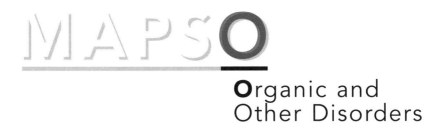

Organic and
Other Disorders

O

Cognitive (Organic) Disorders and Geropsychiatry

■ Cognitive Disorders and Geropsychiatry and the General Clinician

The essential information for the general clinician regarding geropsychiatry includes recognizing the comorbidity and co-occurrence of delirium, depression, and dementia in the elderly population (i.e., "the 3 D's of geropsychiatry"); understanding the risk factors associated with delirium, especially anticholinergic medications, and other adverse reactions to medications; and knowing the basic treatment and management strategies for dementia, agitation, delirium, and late-life depression.

■ Essential Concepts and Terms

Within the MAPSO (mood, anxiety, psychosis, substance, and organic) organizational system, cognitive disorders fall under "O" for "organic." Though the term "organic brain syndrome" is not used within the DSM-IV, it is still in common use to refer to any collection of symptoms that are caused by the direct physiological effect of another general medical condition. Other similar, nonspecific terms include "encephalopathy" and "altered mental status." These terms all refer to global brain dysfunction and may include disturbances in cognition, mood, behavior, consciousness, and thought. DSM-IV cognitive disorders include dementia, delirium, and amnestic disorders.

The 3 D's of Geropsychiatry

When an older patient presents with new symptoms, including a disturbance in cognition, mood, behavior, consciousness, or thought, the diagnosis is often not obvious. An accurate diagnosis may not be made because the symptoms are missed or misattributed to another medical disorder. The early clinical presentations of depression, delirium, and dementia (the 3 D's of geropsychiatry) can sometimes be very similar within the elderly, and it is not uncommon for patients to have 2 or even all 3 simultaneously, as discussed in this chapter.

O

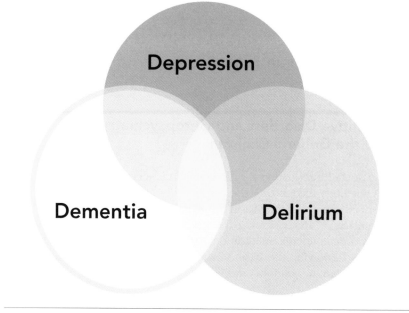

Figure 13-1

Epidemiology

The combined prevalence of cognitive disorders is 15% to 20% in medical inpatients, rising to 50% to 75% in those over 65 years of age. Dementia is primarily a disorder of the elderly, and while delirium can occur at any age, it is most common in elderly medical and surgical inpatients. Since the fastest growing demographic group in the United States is people over 80 years old, geriatric services, particularly geropsychiatric services, will be in high demand over the next 25 years. Much of this need will fall on the shoulders of general clinicians.

■ Dementia

Dementia involves diffuse dysfunction in cognition and other brain functions that is usually progressive. While dementia primarily occurs in the elderly and its incidence increases significantly over age 65, it can occur at any age, even (very rarely) in children. The prevalence of dementia in community residents over age 65 is 5% to 10% but rises to at least 20% in those over age 80. In nursing homes the rate depends on the nature of the home and ranges from 30% to 100%. In general medical inpatients the rate is about 10% to 20%. While most dementias are progressive, some may be static or even reversible.

As with delirium, a mental status exam is the most sensitive (and cost-effective) screening test. Even an extremely brief screen composed of a 3-item recall test and a clock-drawing test (i.e., MiniCog) has excellent sensitivity and specificity (see Screening for Dementia later in this chapter). Memory impairment is required for the diagnosis of dementia, but a variety of neuropsychiatric symptoms may be present, including language disturbances, apraxias (i.e., inability to carry out activity despite intact motor function), agnosia (i.e., failure to recognize or identify the familiar), and disturbances in executive functioning (e.g., planning, organizing, abstract reasoning). Typically patients gradually experience difficulty performing the more complicated activities of daily living, including the ability to work, shop, cook, drive, or pay bills. Poor judgment and lack of insight are common. Psychiatric symptoms are also very common in dementia, including depression, irritability, behavioral disturbances, impulsivity, agitation, hallucinations, and delusions (see Table 13-1).

How extensive an evaluation should be pursued when looking for the etiology of the dementia depends on the particular patient. In the elderly, Alzheimer disease and vascular dementia account for the great majority of cases. Neuroimaging is generally not considered reliable for differentiating Alzheimer disease from vascular dementia, because computed tomography (CT) scans or magnetic resonance imaging (MRI) will typically show brain atrophy with wider cortical sulci and larger cerebral ventricles in most forms of dementia. Alzheimer and vascular dementia frequently occur together. Furthermore, differentiating them has no current substantive therapeutic implications. In young adults, the

Table 13-1 Frequency of Neuropsychiatric Symptoms in Dementia

Delusions	28%
Apathy	21%
Aberrant motor behavior	21%
Irritability	20%
Depression	18%
Hallucinations	16%
Agitation/aggression	16%
Anxiety	15%
Disinhibition	10%
Any 1 of the above	68%

Data adapted from Steinberg et al (1).

Box 13-1 Etiologies of Dementia

Degenerative
- Alzheimer disease
- Dementia with Lewy bodies
- Frontotemporal dementia
- Parkinson disease
- Huntington disease

Vascular dementia (e.g., multi-infarct dementia)

Substances of abuse (e.g., Korsakoff dementia, inhalants)

Medications (e.g., sedatives, anticholinergics)

CNS infection (e.g., HIV, tertiary syphilis, Creutzfeldt-Jakob disease)

Traumatic (e.g., subdural hematoma)

Metabolic (e.g., severe endocrinopathy, B vitamin deficiencies)

CNS neoplasm (e.g., primary or metastatic)

Normal-pressure hydrocephalus

most common causes of dementia are brain injury, alcohol dependence, and HIV/AIDS (see Box 13-1).

Anticholinergic Medications: Association with Dementia and Delirium

Low acetylcholine levels are associated with Alzheimer dementia and delirium. Furthermore, acetylcholine levels decline with age. Many medications' significant anticholinergic properties are well recognized (e.g., diphenhydramine, oxybutynin, amitriptyline), but many other medications have some anticholinergic properties that are not significant individu-

> **Box 13-2 Selected Medications with Anticholinergic Properties**
>
> Amitriptyline (all TCAs)
> Benzotropine
> Codeine
> Colchicine
> Diazepam
> Digoxin
> Diphenhydramine
> Meperidine
> Olanzapine
> Oxybutynin
> Paroxetine
> Prednisone
> Warfarin

ually (e.g., prednisone, olanzapine, meclizine) but are significant when added together. The more drugs with anticholinergic activity a patient is taking, the greater the likelihood of agitation, delirium, and confusion (see Box 13-2).

Case-Finding Strategies

The major considerations in the differential diagnosis of dementia are delirium, depression, and normal age-related changes in memory.

Dementia vs Delirium
While delirium and dementia both include cognitive dysfunction and confusion and both can cause hallucinations, delusions, and incontinence, delirium is distinguished by acute onset, fluctuating course, and the presence of alteration in consciousness. However, delirium and dementia frequently coexist because demented patients are more vulnerable to developing delirium even with minor infections or minor surgery.

Dementia vs Depression
In pure and fully developed form, depression can usually be distinguished from dementia by standard diagnostic criteria. In depression a mood disturbance predominates with much less cognitive dysfunction than in dementia. For example, older patients with major depression are more likely to complain of memory problems because of awareness of cognitive deficits, whereas patients with dementia are typically unaware of their cognitive deficits. Depressed patients tend to complain more and answer mental status questions with "I don't know" or do not answer at all. Demented patients have less insight and awareness and give erroneous answers to mental status questions. Patients suffering from early dementias typically

have intact social skills and use these to cover up when they do not know an answer. It is common for confusion to worsen in the evening. Patients with dementia usually do not complain of their cognitive deficits; rather, their loved ones do. Disorientation, incontinence, and gait problems are not attributable to depression.

The problem is that overlapping syndromes are extremely common. The differentiation of depression accompanied by some cognitive dysfunction, dementia with some depressive symptoms, and coexisting depression and dementia is, at best, very difficult. Depression and dementia share a number of symptoms, including apathy, irritability, emotional lability, sleep disturbance, and anorexia. The diagnosis of depression in a patient known to be demented is also difficult because demented patients generally underreport symptoms due to lack of awareness or language dysfunction, while their caregivers tend to overreport depressive symptoms. The concept of "depressive pseudodementia"—that is, that depression in the elderly can closely mimic dementia—has not been supported by intervention studies. In patients with symptoms of depression and significant cognitive dysfunction, treatment with antidepressants has improved mood and energy, but cognitive dysfunction has remained, which suggests the presence of 2 disorders. In patients with symptoms of both depression and dementia, it may be appropriate to treat empirically with antidepressants and monitor for response in appetite, sleep, affect, and irritability. Anticholinergic antidepressants should generally be avoided because they may increase confusion in patients with cognitive dysfunction (see Anticholinergic Medications: Association with Dementia and Delirium earlier in this chapter).

Dementia vs Age-Related Memory Decline
Like dementia, normal decline in memory becomes more frequent with increasing age. Individuals with normal age-related memory decline (in contrast to most demented patients) are well aware of their deficits. Their answers to mental status exam questions are usually correct, though they may require hints to recall names. Their mood is normal, and they do not have any other symptoms associated with dementia (e.g., aphasia, apraxia, agnosia, or incontinence). The differentiation of dementia from depression and normal age-related memory decline is summarized in Table 13-2.

Table 13-2 Characteristics of Dementia Compared with Those of Depression and Normal Age-related Memory Decline

	Dementia	Depression	Normal Aging
Aware of deficits	No	Yes, complains	Yes
Answers to questions	Often wrong	"I don't know"	Usually correct
Mood	Normal or altered	Depressed	Normal

Screening for Dementia

The current US Preventative Services Task Force (USPSTF) concludes "the evidence is insufficient to recommend for or against routine screening for dementia in older adults" (2). These recommendations are consistent with the American Academy of Neurology (3) and the Canadian Task Force on Preventive Health Care (4) and are based on the lack of evidence that screening all older adults within an unselected population alters the disease course. The USPSTF did find evidence that some screening tests have reasonable sensitivity but only fair specificity in picking up cognitive impairment and dementia; that is, they have limited positive predictive value. This would mean a lot of false positives would result when screening a large, unselected population. However, when evaluating patients who are symptomatic or otherwise thought to be at an increased risk for dementia, the specificity of screening tests would be expected to increase.

The Mini Mental Status Examination is the best-studied instrument for screening for cognitive disorders. The accuracy of the Mini Mental Status Exam is dependent upon the person's age and educational level. Other screening tests—such as the Functional Activities Questionnaire (FAQ), the MiniCog, the Modified Mini Mental Status Examination, the Clock-Drawing Test, the Shore Portable Mental Status Questionnaire, and the 7 Minute Screen—are promising but need further testing in primary care samples. As previously noted, the positive predictive value for these sensitive tests is only fair, but they can be useful in ruling out dementia. Consider a patient population in which the prevalence of dementia is 10% and the positive predictive value of a typical cognitive screening instrument is approximately 40% to 50%. Because the negative predictive value remains over 95%, the screening test may not reliably rule in the diagnosis of dementia, but a negative screening test strongly suggests that dementia can be ruled out.

When a cognitive screening test is suggestive of dementia, one should obtain a collateral history with a focus on functional capacity. Careful questioning of the spouse or other family about the patient's ability to drive, manage a checkbook, pay bills, safely cook, carry out grooming tasks, and perform other activities of daily life will reveal signs of dementia earlier than the diagnosis would otherwise be recognized.

Treatment

The most common reversible cause of dementia is iatrogenic; i.e., the prescription of medications that impair cognitive functioning in the elderly and others who are sensitive to adverse central nervous system (CNS) side effects. Common offenders are anticholinergic medications, sedating antihistamines, opioids, and benzodiazepines.

The younger the patient, the more thorough the search should be for a treatable or reversible cause of dementia, because treatable causes are more frequent in younger patients. In adolescents and young adults who are demented, inhalant abuse should be considered. In older patients for whom Alzheimer disease and vascular dementia are most likely, it is still reasonable to check thyroid-stimulating hormone (TSH), fluorescent treponemal antibody (FTA), B12, and folate levels. In the elderly, imaging studies should generally be reserved for patients who have a history of falls (rule out subdural hematoma), have focal neurological findings on physical examination, or are suspected to have a brain tumor, metastatic cancer, or normal pressure hydrocephalus.

Complications of dementia include depression, psychosis, behavior problems, suicide attempts, feeding difficulties and malnutrition, and incontinence. *Depression in demented patients* should be treated with antidepressants. Start at lower than normal doses because demented patients tend to be more sensitive to CNS side effects. Tricyclic antidepressants should usually be avoided because their anticholinergic properties may exacerbate cognitive dysfunction.

Agitation, aggression, and *psychosis* can cause physical injury as well as psychological morbidity, are upsetting to patients, and are highly stressful for the patients' caregivers. If unmanaged, such behaviors result in nursing home placement, hospitalization, and sometimes longer-term institutionalization. However, agitation is a symptom, not a diagnosis. Agitation should not be treated reflexively with antipsychotics or other medication. The clinician must consider a wide range of possible explanations that are easily missed because the demented patient may not be able to perceive, remember, or communicate the necessary information that would reveal the cause. The patient may be in pain, febrile, delirious, depressed, psychotic, experiencing a medication side effect (e.g., akathisia), or reacting to an environmental change or conflict with (or even mistreatment by) a caregiver.

For many years, *antipsychotic drugs* have been widely prescribed for patients with dementia. Concerns have been raised about overuse of antipsychotic agents to "chemically restrain" patients, particularly in nursing homes. Two recent events have significantly impacted the use of antipsychotic use in elderly patients with dementia. First, the FDA's "black box" warning for all antipsychotics (5), and, second, the initial findings from the CATIE-AD trial showing no benefit for 3 atypical antipsychotics over a placebo (6).

In 2005 the FDA added to all antipsychotics a "black box" warning that said antipsychotics are not approved for dementia-related psychoses, stating, "Elderly patients with dementia-related psychosis treated with atypical antipsychotic drugs are at an increased risk of death compared to placebo." This followed an FDA review of placebo-controlled trials involving the use of atypical antipsychotics in elderly patients with dementia-related behavioral problems. Of the studies included in the FDA analysis, 15 of the 17 trials (including 5106 patients) showed increased numerical death rates associated with olanzapine, aripiprazole, risperidone, and quetiapine (5). (No comparable data on clozapine or ziprasidone use in elderly populations were available, but the FDA mandated that they carry the new warning, too.)

In the Clinical Antipsychotic Trial of Intervention Effectiveness study for Alzheimer disease (CATIE-AD), 421 elderly outpatients with psychosis, agitation, aggression, or Alzheimer-type dementia were treated with a placebo, olanzapine, quetiapine, or risperidone for up to 36 weeks. Rates of improvement did not differ significantly among groups, and the overall discontinuation rates for any reason were 63% after 12 weeks and 82% after 36 weeks.

We urge caution in overinterpreting and overreacting to the CATIE-AD findings or the FDA's "black box" warning. We continue to use these agents within the following parameters:

- Use environmental or behavioral interventions before and after antipsychotics are initiated.
- Use antipsychotics only when clinically necessary (i.e., for psychosis but not as a hypnotic).
- When antipsychotics are used, use them short term at the lowest effective doses.
- Be explicit about the expected outcome for the medication, and, if it is not achieved, then discontinue the antipsychotic.
- Document informed consent, which for psychotic demented patients will be from a family member or other appropriate surrogate decision maker.

Cholinesterase inhibitors may provide some cognitive benefits when initiated early in the course of Alzheimer disease. Their efficacy is considered at best "moderate," and the benefit appears to be in delaying or stabilizing cognitive decline for 12 to 18 months but not in preventing it.

Cholinesterase inhibitors generally have little influence over psychiatric complications of dementia. Limited head-to-head trials between different cholinesterase inhibitors suggest no difference in efficacy. There is further suggestion that any benefits are lost when the drug is stopped (7). A common mistake is the prescription of an anticholinergic drug like diphenhydramine to a patient taking a cholinesterase inhibitor, since any potential benefit is negated. A careful review of medications with obvious and less obvious anticholinergic activity is essential (see Anticholinergic Medications: Association with Dementia and Delirium earlier in this chapter).

The newest drug approved by the FDA for treating dementia is memantine, which has a different mechanism of action. Memantine's demonstrated benefit is a very small reduction of symptoms relative to placebo.

■ Delirium

Delirium typically involves a disturbance in the level of consciousness and cognitive functions developing over a short period of time. The symptoms fluctuate from hour to hour, and often relatively normal moments are interspersed with periods of gross confusion. The level of consciousness may vary from somnolence and stupor to agitation and hyperarousal. Delirious patients are inattentive and easily distractible and are typically disoriented regarding time, place, and the situation they are in. Memory disturbances are common, particularly disturbances in recent memory. Perceptual disturbances include hallucinations or illusions (i.e., misinterpretations of real perceptions). Visual hallucinations are especially common, but hallucinations in all other sensory modalities may occur (i.e., auditory, tactile, olfactory, gustatory). The sleep-wake cycle is disorganized with night-day reversal (i.e., patients tend to sleep during the day and be up at night) and fragmentation of sleep. Emotional lability is common, and a delirious patients' behavior is quite unpredictable. Every ICU is aware that, without warning (and sometimes without awareness), these patients may assault their caregivers and remove tubes and lines. Delirium is easy to spot in the agitated, aggressive, vocally psychotic patient but is often missed in patients with "hypoactive delirium," that is, patients who are quietly confused. The diagnosis of delirium is also commonly missed in children (e.g., their hallucinations are attributed to "normal fantasizing").

Delirium is diagnosed through bedside mental status examination, including testing of patient's orientation, attention, memory, perceptual disturbances, level of consciousness, and behavior. The electroencephalogram (EEG) is almost always abnormal, showing a pattern of diffuse slowing, but the abnormality does not indicate any particular cause of delirium. Other diagnostic tests indicated depend on the patient's history and suspected etiologies, listed in Box 13-3.

Frail, elderly patients, particularly those with dementia or other brain disease, may become delirious with minor infections, such as an uncomplicated urinary tract infection, that would have no such effect in a younger, healthier

> **Box 13-3 Common Etiologies of Delirium**
>
> ---
>
> Medications
> Substances of abuse: intoxication or withdrawal
> Infectious causes
> ■ CNS infections
> ■ Sepsis
> ■ Minor infections (e.g., UTI) in vulnerable hosts
> Metabolic causes
> ■ Electrolyte disturbance
> ■ Vitamin deficiency
> ■ Hypoglycemia
> ■ Hypoxia
> ■ Uremia
> ■ Hepatic encephalopathy
> ■ Severe endocrinopathies
> Traumatic (e.g., brain injury, subdural hematoma, subarachnoid hemorrhage)
> Vascular (e.g., stroke, vasculitis)
> Cancer (e.g., primary CNS, metastatic tumor, paraneoplastic syndrome)
> Inflammatory disorders (e.g., SLE)

person. There is no such thing as "ICU psychosis." Many patients in ICUs are delirious, but their delirium is caused by the diseases or injuries that put them in the ICU (or side effects of the medication or surgery they have received there). The ICU environment itself does not cause delirium, though any unfamiliar environment may be more distressing to delirious patients.

Delirium is associated with significant morbidity and mortality. Patients with delirium stay in the hospital longer and have increased mortality rates both during and after hospitalization. They are likely to extubate themselves and remove other vital lines and tubes. They are uncooperative with treatment and are often impulsively and indiscriminately assaultive toward caregivers. Severe delirium may result in seizures or coma. The intense emotionality, confusion, and fear that many delirious patients experience may result in suicide attempts. Before the introduction of a variety of safety interventions in hospitals, delirium was the most common cause of suicide in medical hospitals. Long-term sequelae of delirium may include post-traumatic stress symptoms and persistent cognitive dysfunction.

Case-Finding Strategies

The differential diagnosis of delirium includes dementia, schizophrenia, and bipolar disorder (see Table 13-3). Malingered delirium is extremely rare. Past history and the setting in which the patient is seen usually point to the correct diagnosis. Delirium is the only one of these diagnoses in which the level of consciousness is altered and the symptoms are usually recent in onset; dementia, schizophrenia, and bipolar disorder are all chronic illnesses. Cognitive dysfunction and incontinence are present in both delirium and dementia but not in schizophrenia and bipolar disor-

Table 13-3 Comparison of Characteristic Features of Delirium, Dementia, Schizophrenia, and Bipolar Disorders

	Delirium	Dementia	Schizophrenia	Bipolar
Consciousness	Altered	Normal	Normal	Normal
Cognitive dysfunction	Present	Present	Absent	Absent
Hallucinations and delusions	Transient, simple	Simple	Persistent, elaborate, bizarre	Persistent, elaborate, mood congruent
Course	New, fluctuating	Pre-existing	Pre-existing	Pre-existing
EEG	Diffuse slowing	Variable	Normal	Normal
Incontinence	Common	Common	Rare	Rare

der. Hallucinations and delusions can occur in any of these, but in delirium and dementia they tend to be simple and not as well-formed or bizarre as they are in schizophrenia. As noted, the EEG in delirium shows diffuse slowing, whereas it is normal in schizophrenia and bipolar disorder and variable in dementia.

There are many different etiologies of delirium (see Box 13-3). The prioritized differential diagnosis of delirium in a 30-year-old alcoholic is different from an 85-year-old nursing home resident, though both could share some of the same potential causes (e.g., pneumonia). One general principle is to identify as quickly as possible those causes requiring emergent intervention.

Treatment

Management of delirium starts with an immediate search for reversible causes. Even if the cause can be identified and rectified, it may take some time before delirium resolves, in which case treatment of the delirium may be required. Treatment is also needed when no reversible cause can be identified.

The first choice of a pharmacologic agent for treating delirium is the neuroleptic haloperidol, which can be given orally, intramuscularly, or intravenously (haloperidol is not approved for intravenous use by the FDA). It is best to start with a very low dose (e.g., 0.5-1 mg every 12 hours) for several reasons. Some patients will respond quite well to low-dose haloperidol. The most common side effects of haloperidol are extrapyramidal reactions, including dystonia and akathisia. The severe sense of restlessness in akathisia may be very difficult to distinguish from the agitation of delirium. Thus, if the dose is too high, the resulting akathisia may be misinterpreted as a sign that the dose is actually inadequate, and the dose is then escalated with poor results. Some brain diseases (e.g., HIV dementia, Lewy body dementia, Parkinson disease) make patients particularly susceptible to extrapyramidal reactions to neuroleptics. Finally, haloperidol can sometimes cause QT prolongation and torsades de pointes. Another reason for keeping the dose of haloperidol as low as possible is that many critically ill patients are already taking other medications that may prolong the QT interval. Having advised starting at a very low dose, we must also point out that there occasionally are patients who have delirium requiring extremely high doses (up to 1000 mg per 24 hours).

Benzodiazepenes generally should not be considered a first choice in the treatment of delirium, except when the delirium is due to withdrawal from alcohol or sedative hypnotics. Many delirious patients with other etiologies respond paradoxically to benzodiazepenes by becoming even more disinhibited and aggressive. For patients who are unable to tolerate an adequate dose of haloperidol, it can often be combined with a short-acting benzodiazepene such as lorazepam, which can also be given orally, intramuscularly, or intravenously. While diazepam can also be as effective as lorazepam, it should never be given intramuscularly because of unreliable absorption.

Environmental and cognitive interventions are often overlooked but are simple and effective. While an unfamiliar environment does not cause delirium, it tends to make it harder for the patient to keep a grip on reality. Patients who normally wear glasses or use hearing aids should have them restored because difficulty with hearing or vision make hallucinations more likely and their understanding of their circumstances less likely. If the patient cannot speak, some other form of communication should be provided. Although physical restraints are currently strongly discouraged by regulatory bodies, they may be essential in many cases of delirium to protect patients from harming themselves or others, as well as from pulling out tubes and lines. In less severely affected patients, providing a 1:1 may provide safety protection and someone who can regularly reorient the patient. As normal a sleep pattern as possible should be promoted. This entails trying to keep the patient awake during the day and avoiding interruptions of sleep during the night. Adequate pain control is very important in the management of delirium, but high doses of opiates may cause confusion, particularly in the elderly. Meperidine should be avoided in delirious patients because it can cause a severe agitated delirium. If medically appropriate, the patient should be encouraged to use a wheelchair or walk. Last but not least, it is very important to explain to patients (even if it appears they cannot understand) and their family that delirium is a temporary state. Both patients and families, particularly when the delirium has included prominent psychotic symptoms and disinhibited behaviors, may fear that the patient has lost his or her mind or has permanent brain damage. Fear of the delirium exacerbates delirium.

■ Late-Onset Depression

The DSM-IV does not have a specific diagnosis of "late-onset depression," but there are some important features of major depression in individuals over 65 that warrant further discussion. The prevalence of major depression in the general population over 65 years of age is estimated to be between 2% and 25%; the latter represents institutionalized patients, and the former represents independent, community-dwelling individuals. When major depression is screened for in the primary care setting, the prevalence is 17% to 34%, and when it is screened for in the general hospital setting, the prevalence of depressive symptoms is 25% to 40%.

Case-Finding Strategies

Precisely defining and diagnosing depression in older adults is difficult because it is hard to distinguish what may be a symptom of depression from a symptom from another cause. Consider a patient with chronic obstructive pulmonary disease (COPD) with decreased concentration, poor sleep, fatigue, and loss of interest in past hobbies who says he feels "depressed" because he now has to wear oxygen all of the time. It is difficult to determine if the somatic symptoms of decreased concentration, poor sleep, and fatigue are related to a depressive disorder or to COPD. It is also not easy to determine whether his or her diminished activity and feeling "depressed" represent a depressive disorder or a normal reaction to COPD's reduction in quality of life. Researchers take an approach either to exclude any symptoms that could be from another cause or to include all symptoms irrespective of cause. We recommend an inclusive approach because it increases the sensitivity of our screening efforts and facilitates early recognition and treatment of depression when present. Using the inclusive approach, the patient in the previous example has a high risk of major depression and should have further assessment to determine what additional management is required.

When assessing a geriatric patient for depression, one of the first tasks is to establish if this is a depressive episode from recurrent major depression or a late-onset depression. Late-onset depression is more likely to have associated symptoms of cognitive decline and psychosis when compared to early-onset depression.

If Major Depression Is Present, Then Screen for Dementia

Growing evidence supports an association between cerebrovascular disease and late-onset depression. A study of a community sample of nondemented elderly found that subjects with white-matter lesions evident on head CT scans were 3 to 5 times more likely to have depressive symptoms than those subjects with normal head CT scans. Further, when patients with late-onset depression (especially patients over 70 years old) are followed over time, they have an increased risk for developing dementia when compared to the nondepressed control subjects. This is especially true for men when compared to women of equivalent age and education (8).

When an older patient (regardless of age) presents with depressive symptoms, it is appropriate and beneficial on several counts to screen with a simple cognitive instrument. First, when a sensitive instrument is used, like the Mini Mental State Examination (MMSE) or MiniCog, and it screens negative for dementia, the clinician can have a relatively high degree of certainty that the patient does not have dementia. If the MMSE is abnormal, then subsequent MMSE scores can be followed over time to measure decline. However, when followed over subsequent years, these patients remain at high risk for developing dementia in the future.

Cognitive symptoms of major depression tend to differ from the cognitive symptoms of dementia. For example, older patients with major depression are more likely to complain of memory problems because of awareness of cognitive deficits, whereas patients with dementia are not typically aware of their cognitive deficits. Other differences in cognitive dysfunction are discussed in more detail earlier in the chapter (see Dementia vs Depression).

Treatment

Most data suggest that late-onset depression is as likely to respond to treatment as early-onset depression. However, given the heterogeneous population of late-onset depression, it is very hard to single out any 1 best agent or approach. Two of the most important things to remember when using antidepressant therapy in the elderly are that *full* doses of antidepressants will be needed just as in younger patients, and that most patients with late-onset major depression who need medication require long-term treatment to maintain remission. The reader is referred to chapters 4 and 5 for discussion of treatments using antidepressant medications.

Psychotherapy

Psychotherapy is as effective in older patients as it is in younger patients and may have particular applicability as an initial treatment for patients with mild-to-moderate depressive symptoms. Most of the evidence in the literature involves cognitive behavioral therapy, but we urge against overinterpreting this as a sign that other psychotherapies, particularly interpersonal therapies and psychodynamic psychotherapies, are ineffective. In general, this cohort has not been studied in enough depth to determine the benefit of one psychotherapy over another, and our experiences suggest that, like younger patients, older patients respond to a variety of approaches when employed by a good psychotherapist.

KEY POINTS

- Dementia, delirium, and depression (the 3 D's of geropsychiatry) tend to co-occur in older patients and should be considered concurrently.
- Screening for dementia should occur in cases in which the likelihood is high, not in every elderly patient.
- Neuropsychiatric symptoms of dementia are common and more effectively treated than the cognitive symptoms of dementia.
- Minimize the number of anticholinergic medications the patient is taking.
- Late-onset depression often predates the onset of dementia.

REFERENCES

1. Steinberg M, Sheppard JM, Tschanz JT, et al. The incidence of mental and behavioral disturbances in dementia: the cache county study. *J Neuropsych Clin.* 2003;15(3):340-345.
2. Screening for dementia in primary care: a summary of the evidence for the US Preventive Services Task Force. *Ann Intern Med.* 2003;138:927-937.
3. Petersen RC, Stevens JC, Ganguli M, et al. Practice parameter: early detection of dementia: mild cognitive impairment (an evidence-based review). *Report of the Quality Standards Subcommittee of the American Academy of Neurology Neurology.* 2001;56:1133-42.
4. Patterson CJ, Gauthier S, Bergman H, et al. The recognition, assessment and management of dementing disorders: conclusions from the Canadian Consensus Conference on Dementia. *CMAJ.* 1999;160:S1-15.
5. US Food and Drug Administration. FDA issues public health advisory for antipsychotic drugs used for treatment of behavioral disorders in elderly patients. FDA Talk Paper T05-13. Rockville, MD: US Food and Drug Administration; April 11, 2005.
6. Schneider LS, Tariot PN, Dagerman KS, et al. Effectiveness of atypical antipsychotic drugs in patients with Alzheimer's disease. *N Engl J Med.* 2006;355:1525-1538
7. Trinh N-H, Hoblyn J, Mohanty S, et al. Efficacy of cholinesterase inhibitors in the treatment of neuropsychiatric symptoms and functional impairment in Alzheimer disease: a meta-analysis. *JAMA.* 2003;289: 210-216.
8. Fuhrer R, Dufouil C, Dartigues JF. Exploring sex differences in the relationship between depressive symptoms and dementia incidence: prospective results from the PAQUID study. *J Am Geriatr Soc.* 2003;51(8):1055-1063.

KEY REFERENCES

Ayalon L, Gum AM, Feliciano L, et al. Effectiveness of nonpharmacological interventions for the management of neuropsychiatric symptoms in patients with dementia: a systematic review. *Arch Intern Med.* 2006;166(20):2182-2188.

Ballard C, Waite J. The effectiveness of atypical antipsychotics for the treatment of aggression and psychosis in Alzheimer's disease. *Cochrane Database Syst Rev.* 2006;1:CD003476.

Boeve BF. A review of the non-Alzheimer dementias. *J Clin Psychiatry.* 2006;67(12): 1985-2001; discussion 1983-1984.

Erlangsen A, Zarit SH, Tu X, et al. Suicide among older psychiatric inpatients: an evidence-based study of a high-risk group. *Am J Geriatr Psychiatry.* 2006;14(9): 734-741.

Fischer C, Bozanovic R, Atkins JH, Rourke SB. Treatment of delusions in Alzheimer's disease-response to pharmacotherapy. *Dement Geriatr Cogn Disord.* 2006;22(3): 260-266.

Inouye S. Delirium in older persons. *NEJM.* 2006;354:1157-1165.

Lacasse H, Perreault MM, Williamson DR. Systematic review of antipsychotics for the treatment of hospital-associated delirium in medically or surgically ill patients. *Ann Pharmacother.* 2006;40(11):1966-1973.

Mitchell AJ, Subramaniam H. Prognosis of depression in old age compared to middle age: a systematic review of comparative studies. *Am J Psychiatry.* 2005; 162(9):1588-1601.

Reynolds CF III, Dew MA, Pollock BG, et al. Maintenance treatment of major depression in old age. *N Engl J Med.* 2006;354:1130-1138.

Schmitt FA, Wichems CH. A systematic review of assessment and treatment of moderate to severe Alzheimer's disease. *Prim Care Companion J Clin Psychiatry.* 2006;8(3):158-159.

Selwood A, Johnston K, Katona C, et al. Systematic review of the effect of psychological interventions on family caregivers of people with dementia. *J Affect Disord.* 2007;101(1-3):75-89.

Tune LE. Anticholinergic effects of medication in elderly patients. *J Clin Psychiatry.* 2001;62(21):11-14.

Medically Unexplained Symptoms in Patients with Psychiatric Disorders

■ Medically Unexplained Symptoms and the General Clinician

Patients with psychiatric disorders frequently present in primary care and other medical settings with physical (i.e., medical, somatic) symptoms. In some cases, the physical symptoms are a manifestation of an underlying psychiatric disorder. When a patient presents with unexplained physical symptoms, many clinicians fall into the trap of framing their task as determining whether the symptoms are "physical" or "psychological." This "either-or" approach has several hazards. First, patients can have both psychiatric and medical disorders, and each may be aggravating the other. Second, this approach creates a false dichotomy that fails to integrate the patient's symptoms with their impact on the patient's life. Third, at its worst, the "either-or" approach can result in extensive, inefficient medical work-ups that prove fruitless. This approach can engender destructive statements like, "We couldn't find anything, so it must be all in your head." Such an extreme does not represent typical clinician behavior, but it illustrates the potential hazards of the "psyche-soma" dichotomy. No patient should ever receive a psychiatric diagnosis solely because the medical work-up was negative.

When clinicians encounter a physical symptom that they cannot clearly attribute to either a psychiatric or medical disorder, the best practice is to be straightforward and tell the patient that the cause is uncertain. Further, such uncertainty is common when working up symptoms and understanding the impact the symptoms have on the patient. This broader, more open approach is especially applicable to the somatoform disorders, discussed in the section titled Five-step Clinical Approach to Medically Unexplained Symptoms.

Patients with medically unexplained symptoms (MUS) are common and familiar to clinicians and present a number of challenges. They frequently present with multiple protean symptoms in diverse organ systems. Often the symptoms are atypical both in their description and as part of a pattern with other symptoms. Many patients with MUS seem to have a disproportionate degree of functional impairment. Such patients tend to take up much more of the clinician's time and utilize more health care resources, including more emergency visits, hospitalizations, diagnostic procedures, and treatment interventions than most patients. Many are heavy consumers of alternative and complementary medicine. They can present additional challenges because they often have unusual sensitivities to side effects of medications and other interventions and high rates of nonresponse to standard treatments. All of these factors put considerable strain on the doctor-patient relationship. Unhappy with their medical care experiences, such patients frequently engage in "doctor-shopping."

Fortunately, most patients with some medically unexplained symptoms do not present such difficulties, and not all such patients have symptoms that are accounted for by psychological factors or a psychiatric diagnosis. Some, but not all, patients with MUS have somatoform disorders, discussed later in this chapter. Other symptoms may be best accounted for by other psychiatric disorders with prominent physical symptoms, such as panic disorder, major depressive disorder, or as yet undiagnosed medical diseases.

■ Essentials Concepts and Terms

Responses to Illness and the "Sick Role"

There is wide variation in how patients experience, respond to, and communicate about their illnesses, affected by culture, socialization, family, and personal experience and traits. Sociologist Talcott Parsons described the "sick role" as allowing persons to be exempted from their normal social obligations and responsibilities (e.g., work, family, school) without blame. Some patients are too ready to embrace the sick role, they fall too far into it, or they are resistant to giving it up when it is time to do so. This may be the result of a number of different psychosocial factors, for example, relief in escaping an abusive relationship or stressful job, a learned pattern of somatizing in one's family, or an abusive or neglected childhood in which the only time the child experienced affection was when he or she was ill. In a normal response to illness, taking on the sick role is adaptive and not pathological. Indeed, refusal to enter the sick role when one should (e.g., continuing to work while denying the symptoms of coronary disease even after having had a myocardial infarction) often represents a maladaptive psychological response. In all of the somatoform disorders discussed later in this chapter, patients have become too attached to the sick role and display a variety of abnormal illness behaviors (e.g., doctor-shopping).

Somatization

The word "somatization" is used in several differing but overlapping ways, but in general it refers to the tendency to experience and communicate psychological or social distress in the form of somatic (i.e., physical) symptoms, which are misattributed to a nonpsychiatric medical cause. Somatization can range from transient to chronic, and it can be a normal response to stress, a culturally determined form of expression, part of a somatoform disorder, or part of other psychiatric disorders (e.g., affective, anxiety, psychotic). Somatization can even be iatrogenic when the clinician is too ready to perceive the patient's distress only in terms of medical disease and launches into a long, fruitless diagnostic and treatment chase. Patients who somatize tend to overperceive and overreact to normal (and abnormal) bodily sensations. This has been termed "somatosensory amplification," which includes general hypervigilance to bodily sensations, selective focus on and magnification of certain sensations, and cognitive and emotional reactions that intensify the sensations and make them more alarming. Many patients with somatization are less likely than nonsomatizing patients to acknowledge that stress or stressors may influence their physical symptoms. This distinction is helpful when interviewing a patient with unexplained medical symptoms because if a patient is absolutely unwilling to consider that "stress" may be contributing to his or her symptoms, then the clinician should consider that some degree of somatization is likely present.

Five-Step Clinical Approach to Medically Unexplained Symptoms

There are 5 basic guiding principles in conceptualizing an approach to the patient with medically unexplained symptoms. First, in patients presenting with somatic symptoms, the initial exclusion of a medical explanation does not per se allow one to infer that the symptoms are psychologically explained. Our ability to reliably exclude medical causation is far from perfect. Diagnosing by exclusion fosters "either-or" thinking, which causes clinicians to overlook the possibility that the patient may have both medical and psychological causes contributing to their symptoms. To diagnose a psychiatric disorder, there should be some affirmative evidence of psychological dysfunction.

Second, even when patients have disorders that are clearly recognized as medical, organic disease pathology often does not adequately account for the magnitude of somatic symptoms and the consequent impairment. Symptom amplification is a common feature of somatization. Clinicians should remember that finding a medical explanation for symptoms does not exclude the possibility that the patient also has a psychiatric disorder contributing to physical symptoms of a medical disorder.

Third, asking whether a symptom is medically caused or psychogenic is undesirable because it fails to recognize the biological, psychological, and social factors in interaction that often contribute to illness. Avoiding the potential hazards of the "psyche-soma" dichotomy allows the clinician and the patient to remain open to all factors that could influence the patient's symptoms.

Fourth, the approach to patients with unexplained medical symptoms should be multidimensional, taking into account the severity of symptoms, the degree of functional impairment, chronicity, comorbidity, and the extent of health care utilization. How the patient has reacted (or overreacted) to his or her symptoms and how much of an impact (proportionate or dispro-portionate) the symptoms have had on him or her are better indicators of somatization than trying to pin down etiologies or biopsychosocial influ-ences.

Finally, the tendency to somatize—that is, to express psychological dis-tress through physical symptoms—exists along a continuous spectrum from normal to highly pathological. Though the normal individual may get "sick" on Sunday night because of anxiety about a presentation at work on Mon-day, the individual with pathological somatization expresses his or her stress through physical symptoms most of the time.

■ Somatization Disorder

Somatization disorder (SD) is at the severe, pathological end of the soma-tizing spectrum. Patients with SD present with a history of multiple physi-cal symptoms for many years, with onset usually as a teenager but always before the age of 30, which leads to seeking care from multiple clinicians simultaneously, doctor-shopping, polysurgery, and polypharmacy. This is the patient classically known as having a "positive review of systems." The somatic symptoms may be vague but usually are dramatic and exaggerated. Concurrent interpersonal dysfunction is usually present. Substance abuse, depression, anxiety, and personality disorders (especially histrionic person-ality) are common. These are patients who are addicted to the sick role.

Symptoms may wax and wane, but the patient tends to remain chroni-cally ill. Epidemiologic studies have found a prevalence of SD in the com-munity of 0.1% to 0.5%, but SD patients account for a much larger and disproportionate share of visits to primary care and other clinicians. Multi-ple factors contribute to the etiology of SD (1,2). Most patients with SD have a history of a chaotic abusive childhood in which early sick-role expe-riences represented rare intervals in which they received care and nurtu-rance. There appears to be a genetic contribution as well, with an increased rate of alcoholism and antisocial personality disorder in male relatives and histrionic personality disorder in female relatives of patients with SD.

Complications include iatrogenic adverse consequences of excessive diagnostic procedures and overtreatment, substance abuse (particularly of prescribed drugs), and suicidal threats and gestures. One significant risk is missing a new medical illness because, like "the boy who cried wolf," the patient has presented with many symptoms so many times before with-out serious medical pathology. The prognosis is poor for a cure, but SD patients can be better managed. Many refuse psychiatric referral and the psychotherapy that could be helpful to them.

Case-Finding Strategies and Management

Important strategies include having one clinician become the patient's main or only doctor, not promising cure, and not scolding the patient. It is also useful to schedule regular, brief outpatient visits on a set schedule that are not contingent on the patient's symptom complaints. At such visits, a focal physical exam should be directed toward whichever symptoms the patient has presented. Laboratory tests, other diagnostic procedures, and treatment should be directed by *signs* rather than symptoms of disease. These strategies have been demonstrated to reduce unnecessary health care utilization and expenditures while maintaining SD patients' health status and actually improving patients' satisfaction. It is important to recognize that the reinforcement of attribution of their symptoms to physical illness sometimes originates from clinicians intently pursuing their investigations for organic disease and ignoring the signs of SD.

■ Conversion Disorder

Patients with conversion disorder develop neurologic symptoms or deficits that do not conform to known pathophysiology or are grossly disproportionate to it. Conversion disorders are thought to arise out of unconscious psychological conflicts, needs, or responses to trauma. Almost any neurologic symptom may be produced, such as paralysis, weakness, seizures, anesthesia, aphonia, blindness, amnesia, and stupor. Conversion disorder often coexists with neurologic illness, the most common example being epileptic seizures and "pseudoseizures" in the same patient. Conversion symptoms often have unconscious meaning, but this will not usually be apparent in initial encounters. Patients with conversion disorder tend to be very suggestible. Some but not all have a strikingly blasé attitude toward their symptoms (e.g., "la belle indifference").

Conversion symptoms can occur at any age but are most likely in adolescence or early adulthood. New onset of unexplained neurological symptoms in elderly patients without a prior psychiatric history are rarely due to conversion disorder. Some conversion symptoms occur as brief, isolated episodes, but others are chronic and recurrent. Conversion symptoms are usually precipitated by an acute stressor or a current emotional conflict. The prevalence of the disorder has varied culturally and historically. The major task in differential diagnosis is determining whether the patient has a neurologic disorder, conversion, or both.

Sigmund Freud posited that conversion symptoms served to protect the individual from unacceptable feelings or unresolvable conflicts and keep such feelings and conflicts out of conscious awareness. This function of conversion symptoms is referred to as "primary gain." In the case of the patient with conversion disorder, the cause of the symptoms is unknown to the patient, even though the cause may seem obvious to the clinician. Such symptoms often elicit gratifying or protective responses from the environment, referred to as "secondary gain" (e.g., sympathy, release from obligations, or disability payments), which in turn reinforce the symptom. Many individuals with chronic conversion symptoms have a history of having been sexually abused in childhood.

Case-Finding Strategies and Management

The management of conversion symptoms begins with careful assessment; a thorough neurologic and physical examination can often distinguish between conversion disorder and organic neurologic disease without the need for other tests. In some cases, specific studies may be required including imaging, electroencephalogram, and electromyogram. It is never helpful to confront the patient in a negative way. Telling the patient "it's all in your head" or "there's nothing wrong with you" angers the patient, reinforces their insistence that the symptoms are "real," and undermines the doctor-patient relationship. The better approach is to first reassure the patient that serious causes like tumor, stroke, or multiple sclerosis have been ruled out, and then tell the patient that they have a form of benign neurologic dysfunction that tends to be exacerbated by stress. Psychotherapy can be very helpful, and the patient is more likely to pursue it if the clinician takes an encouraging and destigmatizing attitude toward the patient's symptoms.

■ Hypochondriasis

Patients with hypochondriasis are preoccupied with their health, amplify and complain about bodily sensations, and worry unrealistically about serious illness. Preoccupation that "something is wrong" is the core feature of hypochondriasis. It is common for some hypochondriacal patients to overuse medical care, whereas others tend to avoid mainstream medicine. All, however, tend to be avid consumers of fad diets, alternative medicine, over-the-counter remedies, vitamin and other supplements, and information over the Internet. The hypochondriacal anxiety may involve a single organ or multiple organ systems. Hypochondriasis is commonly associated with depression, obsessive-compulsive disorder, and other anxiety disorders.

The onset of hypochondriasis is usually in middle to later life. While some individuals at any age experience brief hypochondriacal reactions (e.g., second-year medical students), true hypochondriasis is usually a chronic condition. It is commonly encountered in medical outpatient settings.

One approach to understanding patients with hypochondriasis is based on the recognition that they overexperience and overinterpret their somatic perceptions. Hypochondriacal anxiety may also be a psychological response to poor self-esteem, loss of control over one's life, loneliness, and unhappiness, in which the patient tries to focus their anxiety on a manageable impersonal threat such as a physical disease. The management of hypochondriasis is similar to that of SD. However, if the patient does also have another comorbid psychiatric disorder, particularly depression or an anxiety disorder, pharmacotherapy and psychotherapy may benefit both hypochondriasis and the comorbid psychiatric disorder.

■ Malingering and Factitious Disorder

Malingering is the conscious feigning of illness to achieve a specific gain such as narcotics, release from military duty, release from jail, victory in a lawsuit, or disability benefits. Malingering is actually uncommon except in addicts, sociopaths, prisoners, and soldiers in wartime. Even in those groups, unexplained medical symptoms are not commonly attributable to malingering.

Factitious disorder with physical symptoms (sometimes called Munchausen syndrome) is the intentional, devious production or feigning of medical illness for the primary purpose of imposture (i.e., fooling the clinician or other health care providers). The patient may mimic illness through their recitation of classic history and symptoms, through manipulation of diagnostic tests, or by actually inducing pathology. Patients with factitious disorder often travel from hospital to hospital. Borderline personality disorder frequently accompanies factitious disorder. Factitious disorder is more common in health care workers or their adult children. A variation on this theme is Munchausen syndrome by proxy, in which a parent produces or feigns illness in a child.

Factitious disorder is not common, but it is not as rare as once thought. It is seen most often in tertiary care settings. Although some individuals only produce feigned illnesses intermittently, others persist in a chronic, recurrent, lifelong pattern. This is the most difficult somatoform disorder to diagnose because the patient may manifest no abnormal psychological symptoms on the surface. The diagnosis is usually made by detective work. As with the other somatoform disorders, confrontation is not constructive. Early psychiatric consultation may be helpful in managing the patient, but very few are willing to admit their problem and accept psychiatric treatment.

■ Disability and Its Evaluation

Somatoform disorders are frequent causes of disability (e.g., missed work, days in bed), rivaling chronic medical conditions like diabetes or arthritis.

Consequently, clinicians are frequently asked by patients, employers, or insurers (private or Social Security) to complete disability evaluations for somatoform patients. Some clinicians reflexively release such patients from work and support their receipt of disability regardless of whether they meet disability criteria (which vary by occupation and insurance policy). While such clinicians feel they are acting out of loyalty to their patients, uncritical support for disability promotes invalidism and chronicity of the sick role. The employer, insurer, and patient each have their own interests; clinicians cannot serve all 3 simultaneously and equally. The same problems arise in school- and work-release evaluations. If the somatoform patient's clinician decides to play this role, he or she should be truthful and inform the patient that filling out disability forms will require a break in confidentiality. If the provision of accurate information to employer or insurer will potentially harm the doctor-patient relationship, the clinician can decline to perform the disability evaluation and recommend an independent examination. In any case, all patients who are unable to work or attend school because of somatoform disorders should be treated, and their disorders usually should not be a basis of permanent disability.

KEY POINTS

- Medically unexplained symptoms are extremely common in general practice.
- Asking if the medically unexplained symptoms are "physical" or "psychological" in origin can be misleading for the clinician and the patient.
- The absence of a medical explanation does not by itself allow one to infer a psychological cause, and its presence does not rule out the contribution of psychological factors.
- Pathological somatization involves abnormal health perceptions, thoughts, and behavior with amplified symptoms and attachment to the sick role.
- Somatization disorder is at the extreme end of the somatizing spectrum but can be managed by the general clinician to improve outcomes.
- Conversion disorders are neurological symptoms thought to arise out of unconscious psychological conflicts, needs, or responses to trauma and are best managed though reassurance and psychotherapy.
- The core feature of hypochondriasis is a fearful preoccupation that "something is wrong" with one's body.
- Malingering is the conscious feigning of illness to achieve a specific gain such as narcotics.

- Factitious disorder with physical symptoms (i.e., Munchausen syndrome) is the intentional, devious production or feigning of medical illness for the primary purpose of imposture.
- In a chronically somatizing patient, uncritical support by clinicians for disability promotes invalidism and chronicity of the sick role.

REFERENCES

1. Swartz M, Blazer D, George L, Landerman R. Somatization disorder in a community population. *Am J Psychiatry.* 1986;143:1403-1408.
2. Abbey SE. Somatization and somatoform disorders. In: Levenson JL, ed. *The American Psychiatric Publishing Textbook of Psychosomatic Medicine.* Washington, DC: American Psychiatric Publishing, Inc; 2005:271-296.

KEY REFERENCES

Barsky AJ. Clinical practice. The patient with hypochondriasis. *N Engl J Med.* 2001;345(19):1395-1399.

Ford CV. Decception syndromes: factitious disorders and malingering. In: Levenson JL, ed. *The American Psychiatric Publishing Textbook of Psychosomatic Medicine.* Washington, DC: American Psychiatric Publishing, Inc; 2005:297-310.

Kroenke K, Rosmalen JG. Symptoms, syndromes, and the value of psychiatric diagnostics in patients who have functional somatic disorders. *Med Clin North Am.* 2006;90:603-626.

Mayou R, Kirmayer LJ, Simon G, Kroenke K, Sharpe M. Somatoform disorders: time for a new approach in DSM-V. *Am J Psychiatry.* 2005;162(5):847-855.

Smith RC, Gardiner JC, Lyles JS, et al. Exploration of DSM-IV criteria in primary care patients with medically unexplained symptoms. *Psychosom Med.* 2005;67:123-129.

Smith RC, Lein C, Collins C, et al. Treating patients with medically unexplained symptoms in primary care. *J Gen Intern Med.* 2003;18(6):478-489.

O

15

Personality Disorders

■ Personality Disorders and the General Clinician

Our personalities start to form during childhood, continue to develop through adolescence, and coalesce into a consistent pattern that is sustained throughout life. Personality is the outward projection (i.e., mask) of our internal, individualized patterns of perceiving and processing information, feelings, and experiences. Thus we all develop our individualized styles of coping, and our style (i.e., personality) normally remains consistent throughout our lives. People with healthy or "adaptive" personalities, regardless of style, are flexible when confronted by a stressor; if the first manner of coping does not work, then alternative modes are generated from among an extensive repertoire of coping strategies. Those with personality disorders have very inflexible, and therefore maladaptive, internal coping strategies that they perceive as normal. Personality disorders are thought to arise through the interaction of genetic vulnerability and life's shaping events, particularly early interpersonal experiences. The DSM-IV defines personality disorder as "an enduring pattern of inner experience and behavior that deviates markedly from the expectations of the individual's culture" and results in clinically significant distress or impairment in social, occupational, or other important areas of functioning.

Personality disorders occur in the general population at rates that vary between 10% to 15% but occur in primary care populations at twice those rates (20%-30%). In psychiatric outpatient settings the rate rises to 50%. Clearly, patients with personality disorders seek care from all types of clinicians. Despite the high prevalence, however, most personality disorders go unrecognized or are misunderstood and misdiagnosed.

The "essential" information for the general clinician regarding personality disorders includes the following:

- Knowledge and understanding of personality disorders and their different types and clusters (A, B, and C)
- Common comorbidities found with personality disorders
- Relative magnitude of the personality disorder and the general clinician's countertransference when labeling a patient as "difficult"
- Basic management strategies used in treating personality disorders

■ Essential Concepts and Terms

In the clinical setting, the sooner clinicians realize that they are communicating with someone who has a personality disorder, the better. The interaction between the clinician and a patient with a personality disorder is frequently preceived by the clinician as awkward and uncomfortable. Communication becomes distorted by misperceptions and different expectations from both the clinician and the patient with the personality disorder. What sustains the distorted pattern of communication is the mutual lack of awareness of the other's perception of the doctor-patient relationship. The patient with a personality disorder can only see and experience the interpersonal interactions rigidly. For the patient with a personality disorder, the communication feels "normal" (in the sense of expectable, not pleasurable) because this is what always happens. The self-aware clinician will feel uncomfortable and that something is amiss. Though the clinician's emotional experience in relating to a patient with a personality disorder is often a negative one, positive feelings may be evoked, including paternalistic concern, pity, appreciation of being admired, and even sexual arousal (see Countertransference later in this chapter). In any case, the awkward and tangled style of communication continues for as long as clinicians remain unaware that they are interacting with a patient with a personality disorder. The first step to end this dysfunctional interaction and engage in effective, healthy communication is for clinicians to realize that what they are saying is being misperceived and misunderstood by the patient and to assess the patient for a personality disorder.

Maintaining clear boundaries within the clinician-patient relationship is key in the management of patients with personality disorders. We assume a basic understanding of these boundaries in this chapter. For the reader who wants to review the topic of clinician-patient boundaries, sources are recommended in the references at the end of this chapter.

The 4 E's

It is easier to become aware of a personality disorder in a patient if the clinician knows the general diagnostic features that *all* disordered personalities possess. The DSM-IV's general diagnostic criteria for any personality disorder assume that the individual has a long-standing manner of interacting with others that produces tension and dysfunction, resulting in poor relationships and hampering work and social interactions. To aid in remembering the general criteria for any personality disorder, we use a mnemonic device, "the 4 E's":

- *Early*: The symptoms appear early in adulthood or adolescence.
- *Enduring*: The symptoms endure throughout life.

- *Ego-syntonic*: The manner of interacting with other people is not recognized as abnormal by the person with a personality disorder. Avoidant personality disorder is one exception because it is characterized by prominent anxiety associated with maladaptive behaviors, which frequently cause patients to feel disturbed by their own symptoms.
- *Externalization* of conflict: The intensity of the maladaptive style of a patient with a personality disorder increases under stress. This increases the likelihood that people around the patient will respond in ways that reinforce the maladaptive coping strategy of the person with a personality disorder.

Externalization typically leads to a 5th "E" that stands for *everyone else* other than the person with the personality disorder. Everyone else is typically blamed for causing the stress experienced by the patient with a personality disorder, and everyone else experiences the discomfort that the patient avoids with his or her maladaptive behaviors.

The 3 Clusters and the 10 Personality Disorders

If the patient's style of interacting meets the general diagnostic criteria (i.e., the 4 E's), then that individual most likely has a personality disorder. Of those people who meet diagnostic criteria for a personality disorder, 60% will meet criteria for at least 1 other personality disorder. In other words, "pure" personality disorder types are less common than a mixtures of the types. With this high degree of overlap between personality disorders in mind, it is clinically more effective, efficient, and important to consider which type it may be. The 10 personality disorders are divided into 3 clusters, and each cluster has predominant features that help distinguish it from the other clusters (see Table 15-1 later in this chapter). For the general clinician, recognizing the style and predominant features of each cluster facilitates early awareness and, ultimately, recognition of the personality disorder if present. The following descriptions of each personality disorder are provided as illustrations to help clinicians recognize when they have encountered a patient with a personality disorder. Keep in mind that an individual patient may have characteristics of more than one personality disorder.

Cluster A (Odd, Eccentric)
Paranoid Personality Disorder
These individuals have pervasive distrust and suspicion of others and typically believe that others, including their treating clinician, are exploiting or deceiving them. Full disclosure about the reasons for certain tests or treatments helps minimize their tendency to search for hidden meaning in remarks or actions that others perceive as benign.

Schizoid Personality Disorder
Patients with schizoid personality disorder try to stay socially and emotionally detached from others, avoiding any close relationships and living their lives as much as possible in a solitary fashion. They are uncomfortable with what feels to them like the relative intimacy of medical outpatient and inpatient settings. They do not readily open up to their clinicians and so may not communicate vital information or ask important questions of their doctors. Since they are indifferent to the praise or criticism of others, it is more difficult for health care providers to influence their health behaviors.

Schizotypal Personality Disorder
Patients with schizotypal personality disorder have marked eccentricities that present as odd beliefs or magical thinking. Their vague and sometimes circumstantial speech may seem very anxious. However, the content of the conversation is about odd or highly idiosyncratic perceptual experiences or bodily illusions. It is best not to confront these ideas as "wrong" or "unfounded" but rather offer diagnosis and treatment in parallel with the odd beliefs. However, if the behaviors or beliefs are interfering with treatment (e.g., the patient will not take any pills that are colored, fearing "toxic reactions") or causing significant medical problems (e.g., frequent ear infections because of cleaning with a Q-tip dipped in bleach), then gentle confrontation and redirection is warranted. Also, make sure that the odd beliefs are not part of psychosis from another disorder (e.g., schizophrenia, depression with psychosis).

Cluster B (Dramatic, Emotional)
Antisocial Personality Disorder
Individuals with antisocial personality disorder (ASPD) demonstrate a pervasive pattern of disregard for the rights of others and the rules of society, including the rules and norms of the patient-clinician relationship. Clear, explicit communication about expectations and rules with resultant consequences for violations (e.g., no longer prescribing controlled substances, terminating treatment) is often required. Inappropriate drug seeking and disability seeking can provide early cues to ASPD.

Borderline Personality Disorder
Patients with borderline personality disorder have unstable and intense interpersonal relationships, including those with their health care providers, and their moods swing between overly positive idealization and angry denigration or feeling abandoned. Problems with impulse control that are potentially self-damaging (e.g., impetuous sexual activity, substance abuse, reckless driving) precipitate many of the patient's problems. The general clinician should try to provide a steady and consistent pattern of interaction, avoiding both being drawn in to "fix" the patient's problems (i.e., overinvolvement) and being driven away (i.e., abandonment). Establishment of

realistic expectations, boundaries, and limits and (when the patient is willing) early referral to a mental health clinician are key in management.

Histrionic Personality Disorder

Histrionic patients' excessive emotionality and attention-seeking behavior are dramatic and often sexually provocative or seductive, but it is their tendency for vague, melodramatic, and impressionistic speech (e.g., "I feel like someone took a chainsaw to me") that may lead the clinician to miss a diagnosis or misdiagnose. Dramatically expressed physical symptoms often initially lead clinicians into excessive testing, but subsequently, like the boy who cried wolf, the patient's "real" complaints may not be taken seriously. When dealing with histrionic patients the clinician should realize that what is being talked about is often not the problem. Thus the clinician should ask specific questions targeted toward likely diagnoses and be careful not to get pulled off track or into underreacting or overreacting.

Narcissistic Personality Disorder

The grandiose style and requirement for admiration of those with narcissistic personality disorder inspire angry reactions from others, including clinicians. The clinician's task is to not let the patient's exaggeration of their own talents or sense of entitlement interfere with sound medical treatment. Directly confronting the patient's inflated self-perceptions typically results in unpleasant and unproductive exchanges. Instead, an approach that includes redirection with an opening phrase like, "You deserve the benefits of the best care so . . . ," should yield more productive interactions.

Cluster C (Anxious, Fearful)

Avoidant Personality Disorder

The patient with avoidant personality disorder has an unreasonable fear of criticism, extreme social inhibition, and feelings of inadequacy that make interactions very uncomfortable for both the patient and the clinician. The clinician should not be too aggressive but rather should be reassuring in style. Given the high degree of overlap with social phobia, exploration for additional symptoms or past mental health treatment are important.

Dependent Personality Disorder

The individual with dependent personality disorder has an excessive need to be taken care of, combined with a submissive nature and clinging behavior, which may ambush well-intending clinicians. Clinicians should resist assuming responsibility for making decisions for the patient despite the patient's perceived inability to do so. Rather, the general clinician can offer choices between options and facilitate the patient's autonomous decision. Dependent patients resist this approach, but they also need the clinician and wish to please him or her, so they will try to make some decisions. It is a slow process but one that is far better than the needy and clingy behaviors that can also be present. Excessively gratifying the dependent patient's wishes to be taken care of can create an addiction to the doctor's attentions and acute helplessness when the clinician inevitably is no longer able or willing to continue playing that role.

Obsessive-Compulsive Personality Disorder

Perfectionistic, preoccupied with order and control, and therefore inflexible, patients with obsessive-compulsive personality disorder (OCPD) often come to their medical appointments with detailed lists and notes. They are likely to interpret medical advice very literally. They become very upset over minor scheduling or billing errors. Their expectation of ideal outcomes may make them intolerant of less-than-perfect results. While a person can have both obsessive-compulsive disorder (OCD) and OCPD (though this is uncommon), OCPD is not the same as OCD; that is, patients with OCPD do not characteristically have specific obsessions and compulsions.

Personality Type

Personality types or character styles are important to distinguish from personality disorders. Personality types refer to less maladaptive ways of interacting with the world that do not produce the significant functional impairment seen with personality disorders. Like personality disorders, personality types rarely exist in pure forms; instead, they combine and blend with each other. Also, personality types tend to intensify when a person becomes ill. Generally, this intensified character style is less flexible than one's more adaptive, healthy personality type. In a classic paper in 1964, still very applicable today, Kahana and Bibring described 7 personality types encountered in medical practice: dependent, obsessional, histrionic, masochistic, paranoid, narcissistic, and schizoid (1). Table 15-1 outlines some basic features of each type and the responses the clinician may consider.

Comorbidity

Depression frequently co-occurs with all personality disorders. Each tends to aggravate the other. Between 30% and 50% of patients with cluster C personality disorders have major depression at the time of diagnosis. Patients with cluster A personality disorders have been reported to have comorbid depression in as much as 20% of cases. Those with borderline and antisocial personality disorders (cluster B) have comorbid depression 10% to 30% and 10% of the time, respectively. Treating the depression adequately can improve the flexibility and adaptability of the patient with a personality disorder. In some cases, the patient may no longer meet criteria for a personality disorder after the depression has remitted.

The likelihood of comorbid *substance abuse* is increased in all 3 personality disorder clusters. Recent 12-month prevalence rates from the general population in the United States showed that 48% of people with any drug-related disorder and 25% of people with any alcohol-related disorder

Table 15-1 The 7 Personality Types

Personality Type	Features	Clinician Responses
Dependent	Fears threat of abandonment; needy, demanding, and clingy.	Create predictable structure. Schedule regular visits. Reward independence.
Obsessional	Fears loss of control; meticulous, orderly.	Set a routine. Outline options. Allow patient to choose among them. Considering conducting yourself as a consultant to give patient maximum control.
Histrionic	Seductive, melodramatic; motivated by fear of loss of their attractiveness or love.	Avoid extremes of strict formality and too casual friendliness. Rather, articulate clear boundaries and focus conversations on the patient's fears.
Masochistic	Views illness as a punishment; operates as perpetual victim.	Share the patient's pessimism. Consider framing treatment as another burden to bear.
Paranoid	Distrustful, quick to blame; may view medical interaction as exploitative.	Avoid defensive stance by not confronting irrational fears. Rather, acknowledge patient's feelings, yet continue to work with objectivity and a little more distance.
Narcissistic	Can be arrogant and devaluing of clinician in an attempt to ward off their own feelings of imperfection and vulnerability.	Do not confront patient's entitlement. Rather, reframe entitlement as the good care they deserve. Seeking consultation when appropriate can help validate medical concerns.
Schizoid	Socially awkward and aloof, driven by a fear of intrusion into their personal life.	Maintain gentle interest in patient. Respect patient's privacy. Business-like approach with formality can sometimes be perceived as reassuring.

had a personality disorder (see Table 15-2). For many patients with personality disorder, the major focus of treatment is the comorbid substance-related disorder.

Personality Disorders and Suicide

Personality disorders are estimated to have been present in 30% of completed suicides and 40% of attempted suicides. Suicide occurs disproportionately in cluster B personality disorders. The rates of completed suicide in patients with borderline and antisocial personality disorders are 8% to 10% and 5%, respectively. Patients with borderline personality disorder have very high rates of suicide attempts (60%-75%). Self-injurious

Table 15-2 Twelve-Month Prevalence Rates of Comorbid Personality Disorder in the General Population by Cluster and Substance-rated Disorders

	Cluster A	Cluster B	Cluster C	Any cluster
Any alcohol-related disorder	33.2%	57.8%	50.8%	28%
Any drug-related disorder	16.3%	28%	31.4%	48%

and self-mutilating behaviors are common in borderline personality disorder (e.g., cutting oneself) but much of the time do not represent suicide attempts. Cluster C personality disorders account for about 10% of completed suicides, and cluster A personality disorders account for less than 1% of completed suicides.

For individuals with cluster A or cluster C personality disorders, their increased risk for suicide appears due to comorbid psychiatric disorders (predominantly depression and substance abuse) and not from their personality disorders per se. Only cluster B personality disorders (i.e., borderline, histrionic, narcissistic) have an independent, increased risk for more suicide attempts and more completed suicides after controlling for depression and substance abuse.

The "Difficult Patient"

The term "difficult patient" is highly subjective, and its meaning can vary from clinician to clinician. Some clinicians immediately consider a difficult patient as personality disordered; other clinicians never consider personality disorder. In Groves's classic article, "Taking Care of the Hateful Patient," "hateful" (i.e., difficult) patients are described as those patients with whom clinicians are very uncomfortable (2). Making the doctor uncomfortable is not synonymous with having a personality disorder. In other words, not all patients with a personality disorder are difficult for their clinicians, and not all difficult patients have personality disorders. Other types of difficult patients include, for example, the assertive patient who may make the clinician uncomfortable with strong preferences and persistent questions (not uncommonly a patient who is a nurse or doctor); noncompliant patients; patients with psychosis; and drug-seeking patients with substance abuse problems. It is important not to label patients as having a personality disorder just because they are assertive, noncompliant, or otherwise "difficult."

■ Case-Finding Strategies and Management

Screening for Personality Disorder

In most cases, screening strategies are performed to detect disorders that have known effective treatments (i.e., colon cancer, breast cancer, hypertension, diabetes, major depression). In the case of personality disorders, there is no "cure" per se, and treatments focus on minimizing or containing the maladaptive behaviors and thereby reduce the morbidity of the personality disorders for the patient and those who come in contact with the patient (see Management Strategies later in this chapter). So the purpose of screening for personality disorders is to identify patients whose maladaptive behaviors undermine their interpersonal interactions. For the clinician this means that, by recognizing such patients with maladaptive styles of coping and relating, one can avoid being drawn into dysfunctional doctor-patient relationships. While changing personality traits is difficult at best and takes a long time, clinicians can learn to readily avoid being provoked or otherwise drawn into unhelpful, negative responses to patients with personality disorders.

First of all, the clinician has to be aware that there is a dysfunctional interaction and then recognize what pattern of features are present (e.g., odd, eccentric; dramatic, emotional; anxious, fearful), keeping in mind that a patient may well have traits of more than 1 specific personality disorder type.

Countertransference

One important component of a difficult clinician-patient relationship (even if the patient does not have a personality disorder) is the internal reaction the clinician has toward the patient, which is based on the clinician's internal state. This is called *countertransference*. Countertransference can be defined as the clinician unknowingly "transferring" or displacing onto the patient his or her own feelings in reaction to the emotions, experiences, or problems of a person undergoing treatment. This can express itself as a clinician disproportionately liking or disliking a particular patient. In some cases, strong countertransference reactions reflect the clinician's own background, and the patient is only an innocent prompt to the clinician's memories. For example, the patient may remind the clinician of a family member or significant other person with whom the clinician had an intense emotional relationship. It is not "bad" for a clinician to have these feelings; indeed, it is inevitable. But if the clinician remains unaware of the feelings or of their true source, those feelings can distort the clinician's perceptions of and relationship with the patient.

Countertransference reactions to patients with personality disorders are especially likely and strong because the patient's behaviors can be very frustrating, as previously illustrated. This can be a hazardous situation, both because the reactions of the patient and clinician can become mutually inflamed and because the clinician's judgment can become clouded.

When a difficult patient, or any patient, provokes an intense emotional response, the clinician should stop and assess his or her own internal state as it pertains to the patient. This entails asking oneself, *What is it about this patient that is getting to me? Is it something the patient is doing, or is this something about me? Or is it both?*

Management Strategies

The American Psychiatric Association (APA) Practice Guideline for treating borderline personality disorder serves as a good example to guide treatment for all personality disorders. The backbone of treatment is psychotherapy. The APA guidelines do not recommend a particular type but instead cite several different effective psychotherapies. Medications are directed toward comorbid conditions and symptom reduction. No drug therapy has been proven to resolve the personality disorders themselves.

The literature emphasizes that the goal of treatment is care and not cure. Over time, where adaptive corrective interactions are repeated sufficiently, many patients will stabilize and some, particularly those with comorbid conditions that are adequately treated, will improve. Patients with personality disorders present management challenges for any clinician. The general clinician should have a low threshold for referring the patient for psychiatric consultation and psychotherapy.

KEY POINTS

- Personality disorders are twice as common in the primary care setting as in the general population (20%-30% vs 10%-15%).
- Most personality disorders are unrecognized in the primary care setting.
- Remember the "4 E's," the general criteria for any personality disorder:
  - Early: The symptoms appear early in adulthood or adolescence.
  - Enduring: The symptoms endure throughout life.
  - Ego-syntonic: The patient himself is typically not discomforted by his or her personality.
  - Externalization of conflict: Other people experience discomfort around the person with the personality disorder.
- Be aware of the potential for countertransference (displacing your own emotions onto the patient).
- Consider collaborating with another clinician or psychiatrist in the care of the patient with a personality disorder.

■ Treatment for the patient's maladaptive coping strategies relies on psychotherapy. No drug therapy cures the personality traits themselves. Medications are directed toward comorbid conditions and symptom reduction.

REFERENCES

1. Kahana RJ, Bibring GL. *Personality Types in Medical Management, in Psychiatry and Medical Practice in a General Hospital.* Ed. Zinberg NE. Madison, CT: International Univ. Press; 1964:108-123.
2. Groves JE. Taking care of the hateful patient. *NEJM.* 1978;298:883-887.

KEY REFERENCES

Gabbard GO, Nadelson C. Professional boundaries in the clinician-patient relationship. *JAMA.* 1995;273(18):1445-1449.

Gerson J, Stanley B. Suicidal and self-injurious behavior in personality disorder: controversies and treatment directions. *Curr Psychiatry Rep.* 2002;4:30-38.

Gutheil TG, Gabbard GO. The concept of boundaries in clinical practice: theoretical and risk-management dimensions. *Am J Psychiatry.* 1993;150(2):188-196.

Livesley WJ. *Practical Management of Personality Disorder.* New York: Guilford; 2003.

Moran P, Jenkins R, Tylee A, et al. The prevalence of personality disorders among UK primary care attenders. *Acta Psychiatr Scand.* 2000;102:52-57.

Noyes R, Langbehn DR, Happel RL, et al. Personality dysfunction among somatizing patients. *Psychosomatics.* 2001;42:320-329.

Olfson M, Fireman B, Weissman MM, et al. Mental disorders and disability among patients in a primary care group practice. *Am J Psychiatry.* 1997;154:1734-1740.

Skodol AE, Oldham JM, Gallaher PE. Axis II comorbidity of substance use disorders among patients referred for treatment of personality disorders. *Am J Psychiatry.* 1999;156:733-738.

Zimmerman, Rothschild L, Chelminski I. The prevalence of DSM-IV personality disorders in psychiatric outpatients. *Am J Psychiatry.* 2005;162:1911-1918.

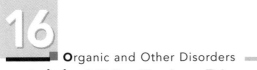

Adult ADD, Eating Disorders, and Women's Mental Health

■ Adult Attention Deficit Disorder

Essential Concepts and Terms

Attention deficit/hyperactivity disorder (ADHD) and attention deficit disorder (ADD) are disorders that have onset in childhood with symptoms falling into 3 general categories: inattention, hyperactivity, and impulsivity.

The DSM-IV criteria further require that the symptoms cause impairment and were present before age 7. The symptoms present in the majority of the cases diagnosed in childhood remain relatively stable until adolescence, when they begin to attenuate. By early adulthood, most people with childhood-diagnosed ADD or ADHD do not require further treatment despite retaining some residual components of the disorder. It is estimated that between 30% and 60% of ADHD patients will retain some symptoms into adulthood. Though the full complement of their childhood symptoms will not be present for most adults, a significant minority will retain symptoms that warrant ongoing treatment.

The symptoms of hyperactivity and impulsivity (i.e., ADHD) impair children's abilities to participate in the classroom and in orderly play and to make friends. Hyperactivity and impulsivity symptoms are more likely to be recognized and treated in childhood and fortunately usually resolve by adulthood. The diagnosis of ADD is more easily missed in childhood, when hyperactivity and impulsivity symptoms are mild or absent and only the symptoms of inattention and distractibility are present. Though the symptoms of inattention and distractibility also attenuate over time, they usually maintain a greater magnitude of intensity than hyperactivity and impulsivity and therefore can continue to cause problems into later life. These patients can present as adults with poor job performance or those not realizing their full potential in their chosen occupations.

Epidemiology

Estimates of the prevalence of ADD and ADHD range from 3% to 10% for school-aged children and from 2% to 4% for adults. Although boys with ADD or ADHD outnumber girls with ADD or ADHD (about 3 to 1), it appears that men and women are equally affected by ADD and ADHD. Genetic studies show that parents of ADHD children have prevalence rates of ADHD of about 40%. Children of ADHD adults have rates of ADHD of around 50%.

Comorbidity

Psychiatric comorbidity in adults with adult ADD is very frequent (see Table 16-1), with substance abuse being the most common, followed by anxiety disorders and major depression.

Case-Finding Strategies

Many patients are not diagnosed with ADD or ADHD in childhood but present as adults. Typically, a young adult will present in his or her middle to late 20s with impairment in work or in relationships. Women may be less frequently diagnosed in childhood because girls tend to have less of the hyperactivity and impulsivity than boys, who behaviorally attract attention and subsequent diagnosis. One group of patients with ADD who present in adulthood is patients with a high IQ and ADD. Individuals with high IQs may be able to compensate for their attention deficits in childhood but then become labeled as underperformers or as "not living up to their potential." Another common scenario is an adult whose child has recently been diagnosed with ADD or ADHD. Frequently adults with ADD and ADHD whose diagnosis was missed in childhood present for treatment with one of the comorbid diagnoses. The clinician should consider whether the evident condition (e.g., alcohol abuse or depression) fully accounts for the patient's inattention and distractibility or whether the patient may also have unrecognized ADD. In such cases, consideration of diagnosis and treatment for ADD should usually be postponed until the evident condition has been treated. In other words, ADD should only be considered if its symptoms persist after resolution of the symptoms of, for example, alcohol abuse or depression.

In order to meet the diagnostic criteria of adult ADD, the individual should have sufficient symptoms to have met the diagnostic criteria for ADD and ADHD in childhood. ADD and ADHD always begin in childhood and never first develop in adulthood. The diagnosis of childhood ADD or ADHD made retrospectively is difficult at best and highly subjective. Collateral history from parents or relatives, school transcripts, and neuropsychological testing can all be helpful. As noted previously, ADD and ADHD

Table 16-1 Lifetime Comorbidity in Adults with ADHD	
Comorbidity	Prevalence in Adults with ADHD
Alcohol abuse	27%-36%
Panic and other anxiety disorders	20%-43%
Major depression	17%-30%
Antisocial personality disorder	12%-18%
Bipolar disorders	5%-10%

tend to run in families. Though a positive family history increases the likelihood of the diagnosis, a negative family history does not change the likelihood of the diagnosis much.

Mimics

Not every patient with a deficit in attention has ADD. Most adults who present to their general clinician with a chief complaint of inattention have a diagnosis other than ADD. Common alternative diagnoses include depression, substance abuse, generalized anxiety disorders (GAD), sleep disorders, learning disabilities, medical causes of fatigue, and normal age-related memory decline.

One of the compelling reasons for diagnosis and treatment of ADD and ADHD in childhood is to potentially prevent a future comorbid disorder. Learning disabilities (LD) also begin in childhood and can go undetected like ADD and ADHD. Like the other disorders mentioned, LD can both mimic and co-occur with ADD and ADHD. Neuropsychological and educational testing can be helpful in teasing these two apart.

Treatment

Management of adults with ADD and ADHD should progress methodically and be handled with patience. While many patients come to their clinicians already convinced they have ADD (e.g., based on Internet checklists, print media, TV shows), jumping right to prescribing a stimulant is seldom indicated because the diagnosis so often is not ADD. Even if it turns out to be the correct diagnosis, the symptoms have been present for the patient's entire life, so the clinician should take sufficient time to find the correct diagnosis or diagnoses and plan appropriate treatment. The first step in treatment of ADD and ADHD is to identify all of the disorders present (e.g., ADD alone, ADD plus depression, ADHD plus substance abuse, ADD plus sleep disorder). As mentioned earlier, in most cases, if a comorbid disorder is present that can cause inattention, it should be treated before a diagnosis of ADD can be fully considered and before initiating stimulants. In some patients, successful treatment of the comorbid disorder will sufficiently reduce inattention and distractibility so that no further treatment is necessary.

The next step is confirming a diagnosis of ADD or ADHD on a basis other than just the patient's current complaints (see Case-Finding Strategies earlier in this chapter). *Some clinicians believe that a positive response to a stimulant specifically confirms the diagnosis of ADHD, but it does not.* In fact, most normal people without ADD will have improvement in their cognitive functioning with the use of stimulants. *A negative response to treatment with a stimulant does not rule out the diagnosis of ADD or ADHD.* About 30% of adults with ADD will not respond to their first stimulant and will require either a dose increase or change to an alternative medication.

Assuming that a diagnosis of ADD or ADHD has been reached and that there are no active comorbid disorders, the next step is to educate the patient about the disorder. Education is exceedingly important because there are frequent misperceptions on the patient's part as to what they can expect from treatment. "A pill will make it all better" is an unrealistic notion that many patients (and some clinicians) have. A more reasonable expectation is that treatment including medication will help the patient be less symptomatic and function better. Given the nature of ADD and ADHD in adults, the symptoms seldom completely disappear with treatment, though they may continue to abate over time and the patient will hopefully experience less dysfunction as well.

Environmental and Behavioral Modifications

Environmental and behavioral changes can provide improvement in the patient's quality of life. Learning strategies for organization, developing routines, and minimizing distractions benefit occupational and social functioning. It is not uncommon for patients with ADD or ADHD diagnosed as adults to change career paths to ones that are more suitable for people who are easily distracted. At the very least, changes in the work and home environments can minimize distractions. For example, it is extremely difficult for someone with ADD or ADHD to work in a cubical where multiple conversations are heard and people frequently walk by. On the other hand, quiet background music may increase attention and not distract them. Educating the patient's family or significant other is also very helpful.

Pharmacotherapy

The options for pharmacotherapy for ADD and ADHD include nonstimulant medications (e.g., atomoxetine, bupropion, desipramine, venlafaxine) and stimulants (i.e., methylphenidate-based stimulants and amphetamine-based stimulants).

Whether to start first with a stimulant or a nonstimulant depends on a number of factors, including patient preference. Some patients have strongly held positive or negative beliefs about a particular drug based on the experience of their children with ADD or ADHD, and such beliefs should be taken into consideration. Some patients do not wish to take stimulants, fearing addiction or because of other negative associations. For a patient with ADD or ADHD and depression, one of the antidepressants effective in treating both disorders (e.g., bupropion, venlafaxine, and desipramine) would be a good place to start. Stimulants should be avoided in patients with a history of substance abuse and are almost never indicated in those who have abused cocaine or amphetamines (though those who abuse should be distinguished from those who may have taken their roommate's Ritalin to see if it would help). As previously noted, substance abuse frequently accompanies ADD or ADHD in adults, and patients with both should be treated by specialists.

Atomoxetine (Strattera) is a selective norepinephrine reuptake inhibitor approved for the treatment of adults with ADD or ADHD. Though the package insert suggests starting at 40 mg and then increasing to 80 mg after 4 days, lower and slower titration reduces side effects. Further increases up to 120 mg per day are sometimes needed. The 2 most common side effects are dry mouth and insomnia. Atomoxetine is a good choice for ADD or ADHD patients with a history of substance abuse because it is not addictive and not a controlled substance.

Treatment with stimulants (in adults without substance abuse or medical contraindications) is relatively safe, and they also carry the greatest effect size for the treatment of ADD and ADHD. The effect size (i.e., the magnitude of difference between the active drug and placebo) for stimulants in treating ADD and ADHD ranges from 0.8 to 0.9. For comparison, the effect size for a selective serotonin reuptake inhibitor (SSRI) in treating depression is 0.35 to 0.4. Response to a given dose of a stimulant is seen within days, while response to nonstimulants usually takes weeks. The major side effects of stimulants include insomnia, gastrointestinal upset, decreased appetite, increased heart rate, elevated blood pressure, and jitteriness. At the doses used to treat ADD and ADHD, stimulants do not typically cause anorexia or weight loss. Stimulants are relatively contraindicated in patients with structural heart disease, uncontrolled severe hypertension, untreated hyperthyroidism, glaucoma, psychosis, and uncontrolled anxiety. Stimulants should not be used by patients who are nursing or who have taken a monoamine oxidase inhibitor within the past 2 weeks.

Stimulants can be initiated in the immediate-release form and then switched to an extended-release form or started in the extended-release form. We find ourselves initiating extended release forms more frequently because they eliminate the switch-over step and also eliminate the "up and down" effects of immediate-release stimulants. While both methylphenidate-based and amphetamine-based stimulants are equally effective, individual patients often respond better to one or the other, and there is no way to determine this other than empirically. As previously noted, 30% of ADD and ADHD patients do not have sufficient results with their first trial of a stimulant. If this occurs, using an agent with a different parent compound is recommended. If a patient has not responded to trials of nonstimulants and methylphenidate-based and amphetamine-based stimulants, a trial of modafinil (Provigil) can be considered, though it is very expensive and this is an off-label use not covered by most insurers. See Table 16-2 for more information.

Table 16-2 Pharmacotherapy for Adult ADD

	Active Compound	Brand Name	Dose	Duration of Action
Amphetamine Based	Dextroamphetamine (Short-acting)	Dexedrine, Dextrostat	5-20 mg	3-5 h
	Dextroamphetamine (Long-acting)	Dexedrine Spansules	20 mg	8-12 h
	Amphetamine/ Dextroamphetamine (Short-acting)	Adderall	5-30 mg twice a day	4-8 h
	Amphetamine/ Dextroamphetamine (Long-acting)	Adderall XR	5-30 mg twice a day	8-12 h
Methylphenadate Based	Methylphenidate (Short-acting)	Ritalin	5-30 mg bid	3-4 h
	Methylphenidate (Long-acting)	Ritalin SR	20-60	4-8 h
	Methylphenidate (Long-acting)	Ritalin LA	20-60 mg	8-12 h
	Methylphenidate (Long-acting)	Metadate CD	20-60 mg	8-12 h
	Methylphenidate (Long-acting)	Focalin XR	10-30 mg	8-12 h
	Methylphenidate (Long-acting)	Concerta	18-72 mg	12 h
Non-stimulant Medications	Atomoxetine	Strattera	25-120 mg	24 h
	Bupropion	Wellbutrin SR	100-400 mg	24 h
	Desipramine	Norpramin	100-300 mg	24 h

■ Eating Disorders

Essential Concepts and Terms

Abnormal eating behaviors (e.g., binging, restricting, purging) and commonly associated symptoms (e.g., distorted body image) can be conceptualized by either a categorical approach (i.e., disorder vs nondisorder) or a dimensional approach (i.e., a spectrum ranging from normal to abnormal). The DSM-IV provides the criteria for each category or disorder: anorexia nervosa (AN), bulimia nervosa (BN), binge-eating disorder (BED), and eating disorder not otherwise specified (EDNOS). These narrow, tight definitions facilitate research that ultimately provides evidence to guide treatments. However, many patients in the clinical setting have abnormal eating behaviors but do not meet all of the criteria required to diagnose a particular eating disorder. Thus the dimensional approach has greater utility for assessment of abnormal eating behaviors.

Approaching each dimension of abnormal eating from nutritional, behavioral, and psychological perspectives allows the clinician to evaluate each component across a spectrum from normal to abnormal. In this section we will discuss the 4 primary eating disorders defined in the DSM-IV, each of the 3 major dimensions (i.e., nutrition, behavior, and psychology), and screening and assessment strategies.

Anorexia Nervosa

Anorexia nervosa (AN) is primarily defined by voluntary restriction of caloric intake despite significant physical consequences associated with malnutrition. It is estimated that about 0.7% of teenage girls in Western countries have AN. It affects 10 females for every 1 male. Though all of the eating disorders vary in severity, AN is associated with mortality rates as high as 5% per decade. Most patients with AN will not "complain" about their low weight. A visit to their clinician may be prompted by amenorrhea, orthostasis, or another medical complication, but the patient will reject advice to increase her weight because she perceives herself as overweight, not underweight. The DSM-IV criteria for AN include the following:

- Refusal to maintain a body weight of at least 85% of ideal body weight
- Intense fear of gaining weight despite being underweight
- Distorted body image
- Amenorrhea in postmenarchal females

Though not required for the DSM-IV diagnosis, many patients with AN will also binge and purge as well as abuse laxatives and diuretics and exercise excessively. In addition to amenorrhea, other physical signs and complications include orthostatic hypotension, hypokalemia, hyponatremia, metabolic alkalosis, bradycardia and other arrhythmias, QTc interval prolongation, low serum albumin, high serum uric acid, osteoporosis, stress fractures, myopathy, gastroparesis, and constipation. Chronic use of ipecac is particularly dangerous, as it can be associated with the development of cardiomyopathy. Vomiting may cause complications related to acid reflux, such as enlargement of salivary glands, dental caries, esophagitis, and gastritis. When patients with AN are given intravenous nutrition, they may develop refeeding hypophosphatemia.

Bulimia Nervosa

Bulimia nervosa (BN) is primarily defined by abnormal eating behaviors involving binges of eating followed by compensatory "purging" activities that include induced vomiting, excessive exercise, and laxative abuse. It is estimated that about 1% to 2% of teenage and young adult women in Western countries have BN. It affects 30 females for every 1 male, but the incidence in males has been increasing in recent years. BN is generally considered to have a more favorable course than AN, even though many patients with BN continue to purge even 10 years after the initial diagnosis. The DSM-IV criteria for BN include the following:

- Recurrent binge eating with a feeling of lack of control of the eating
- Recurrent inappropriate compensatory behavior
- Both of the above occurring, on average, at least twice a week for 3 months
- Distorted body image

As previously noted, AN can include binging and purging behavior, and this may be part of the commonly seen progression from AN to BN. In other words, a patient who has AN with binging and purging can change her behaviors and not restrict food intake and essentially convert to BN. However, patients with BN who are overweight or of normal weight rarely convert to AN. There is growing awareness of BN-like behaviors in type I diabetic women who calorically "purge" by not using insulin. The result is higher blood glucose, more ketosis, and more end-organ complications (e.g., retinopathy). An eating disorder should be considered in any young woman with unexplained, difficult-to-control diabetes.

Binge-Eating Disorder

Binge-eating disorder (BED) is a provisional diagnosis within the DSM-IV, but it does appear to be a discrete and valid disorder. The diagnoses of BED and BN both share binge-eating behaviors; however, in BED there are no compensatory purging behaviors. There are few community-based studies of the prevalence of BED. It does appear to be more common than BN and have a fairly high rate of spontaneous resolution. BED affects 4 females for every 1 male. The DSM-IV criteria for BED include the following:

- Recurrent binge eating with a feeling of lack of control of the eating
- Marked distress regarding binge eating
- Binge eating occurring, on average, at least 2 days a week for 6 months

Eating Disorder Not Otherwise Specified

Eating disorder not otherwise specified (NOS) is the most common of the eating disorders described in the DSM-IV. Its lack of specificity and greater prevalence than the other eating disorders speak to the heterogeneous nature of eating-disordered behaviors. Two syndromes in this category are night eating syndrome and nocturnal sleep-related eating disorder. Night eating syndrome is a disorder in which affected individuals wake multiple times during the night and are unable to fall back asleep unless they eat, and they usually end up binging on high-calorie foods. Nocturnal sleep-related eating disorder is not, strictly speaking, an eating disorder. It is thought to be a type of sleep disorder in which people eat while seeming to be sound asleep. Both are more common than previously thought.

Case-Finding Strategies

Dimensional Approach to Abnormal Eating

Assessing a patient with abnormal eating is accomplished best by exploring her symptoms across 3 dimensions: nutritional, behavioral, and psychological. The nutritional dimension primarily examines the patient's actual weight vs the expected weight. Lower-than-expected weights lead the clinician to inquire more about food restriction; higher-than-expected weights lead the clinician to inquire more about binge eating. Other nutritional parameters (e.g., hypoalbuminemia) may also be cues to the diagnosis. Thus, the nutritional assessment leads to the behavioral assessment of eating (e.g., restricting, binging) and ultimately exploration for compensatory behaviors (e.g., vomiting, excessive exercise). The psychological dimension (e.g., distorted body image) is last, in large measure because it is unlikely to come up in general medical clinical encounters unless nutritional and behavioral abnormalities have been observed and the patient is asked about it. Interestingly, even patients whose AN or BN have resolved nutritionally and behaviorally seldom have complete resolution of their distorted body images.

Screening for Eating Disorders

Most patients with eating disorders will not present for treatment of their abnormal eating behaviors. When directly asked about eating, they may be defensive and evasive, but many will generally answer accurately. The following are examples of good screening questions.

Are you satisfied with your body size?

Does your weight affect the way you think about yourself?

Do you worry that you will lose control over eating?

How many diets have you undertaken in the last year?

The patient's verbal and nonverbal behaviors (e.g., looking away, shifting around) all give the clinician clues about whether to proceed with more questions about eating disorders or to look for other causes for the signs and symptoms present. When a significant eating disorder is detected, consultation with a mental health specialist is indicated.

Treatment

There is not a single formula or algorithm that fits every patient, but early detection, collaborative management, psychotherapy, careful nutritional monitoring, and patience are all part of successful treatments of eating disorders. Treatment of eating disorders is made even more difficult because the patients are often resistant to treatment and in extreme cases go to great lengths to undermine treatment. The first order of treatment is nutritional. This stage focuses on correction of fluid and electrolyte abnormalities, followed by appropriate caloric supplementation in the patient's diet. These measures are ideally carried out in specialized inpatient facilities designed for the specific treatment of eating disorders. In less severe cases the eating disorder is managed in a collaborative manner between mental health professionals and other medical clinicians. Psychotherapy is the primary approach to both AN and BN. There are no proven pharmacologic remedies for AN, though antidepressants are helpful for comorbid depression or OCD. Studies are mixed regarding the value of antidepressants in BN, though antidepressants can be helpful with comorbid depression. In any case, except for the mildest forms of these disorders, the general clinician should not attempt to treat without a mental health professional in collaboration.

■ Women's Mental Health

Premenstrual Dysphoric Disorder

During the late luteal phase of menstruation, up to 75% of women experience some mood, behavioral, or somatic symptoms. Between 20% and 50% of menstruating women have severe enough symptoms to be considered to have premenstrual syndrome (PMS). However, as Figure 16-1 demonstrates, most women with PMS do not have sufficient severity of symptoms or functional impairment required to diagnose a disorder such as premenstrual dysphoric disorder (PMDD) (see Box 16-1). Though there has been skepticism about the existence of PMDD, it has been rigorously and prospectively verified. The DSM-IV characterizes PMDD as marked depressed mood, marked anxiety, emotional lability with premenstrual onset, and remission of symptoms shortly after the onset of menses. PMDD will only affect about 3% to 8% of menstruating women.

The clinical challenge for the general clinician is distinguishing other psychiatric disorders that may be exacerbated during the luteal phase from PMDD. Mood disorders (e.g., major depression, dysthymia) and anxiety disorders (e.g., GAD) are common in menstruating women. In a study of women who presented to a specialty clinic with self-identified PMS or

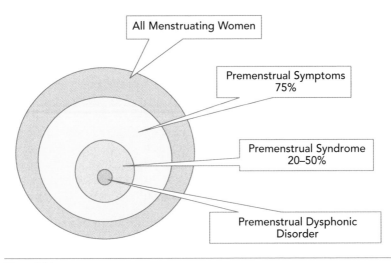

All Menstruating Women

Premenstrual Symptoms
75%

Premenstrual Syndrome
20–50%

Premenstrual Dysphonic
Disorder

Figure 16-1

PMDD, 40% were subsequently diagnosed with either a mood disorder or an anxiety disorder. The patient's report of having only premenstrual symptoms is often a misperception. Rather, there are unrecognized symptoms present earlier in the menstrual cycle and then premenstrual intensification of symptoms. Before the diagnosis of PMDD is given, at least 3 prospective cycles should be observed. A diary is helpful for this task, targeting the major symptoms (e.g., irritability, depressed mood, physical symptoms) and tracking them throughout the entire menstrual cycle and not just the premenstrual part. PMDD, like other premenstrual symptoms, abates after menopause.

Most women with PMDD do not present for treatment; instead they use complementary and alternative medicines (CAMs) at very high rates. One PMS clinic reported that 91% of their patients

Box 16-1 Criteria for PMDD

Five or more of the following symptoms must have been present during the last week of the luteal phase, with at least 1 being from the first 4:

1. Feeling sad, hopeless, or self-deprecating
2. Feeling tense, anxious, or "on edge"
3. Marked lability of mood interspersed with crying
4. Persistent irritability and anger, increased interpersonal conflict
5. Decreased interest in usual activities, social isolation, and withdrawal
6. Difficulty concentrating
7. Fatigue and lethargy
8. Hypersomnia or insomnia
9. Subjective feeling of being overwhelmed or "out of control"
10. Physical symptoms of being bloated, breast tenderness, or weight gain with tightness of clothes fitting

This pattern must have existed most months for the preceding 12 months. The symptoms disappear shortly after the onset of menses.

used CAMs and 53% reported that they helped. This is despite a paucity of scientific support for these approaches. There is some evidence that vitex agnus castus (chasteberry) may be beneficial. First-line treatment for PMDD is usually an SSRI at usual dosage either given continuously throughout the cycle or just during the luteal phase (i.e., starting at ovulation and stopping with the onset of menses). Both approaches produce responses that are statistically superior to a placebo. Hormonal therapies that produce an anovulatory state are used as a second line of treatment for patients who fail SSRI treatment. Gonadotropin-releasing hormone (GnRH) agonists have comparable results to SSRIs. Hormonal therapy seems to have a greater effect on the physical symptoms than the psychiatric symptoms, and SSRIs have a greater effect on the psychological symptoms than the physical symptoms. However, both lines of treatment have effects on both types of symptoms.

Psychiatric Medications in Women of Childbearing Years

Weighing the risks and benefits of psychiatric medications in women contemplating pregnancy is very important and challenging. It is important because all potential options carry some risk (including foregoing medication), and it is challenging because the evidence is complex and not easily explained so that the patient can make an informed decision. The focus of this process is on balancing the risks to the fetus or baby vs the risks to the mother while recognizing that there is the risk of potential harm to the fetus or baby with all options.

When discussing the risks with patients, it is best to discuss risk in terms of changes in absolute risk instead of changes in relative risk. For example, Ebstein anomaly occurs in about 1 in 20,000 births (0.005%) and 1 in 1000 births (0.1%) of women taking lithium. The change in relative risk is 20-fold, but the change in absolute risk is <0.1%. Given that the baseline risk for any abnormality is between 3% and 4%, the impact of lithium on the risk for Ebstein anomaly is very small. However, if a baby is born with Ebstein anomaly, then the discussion of risk will have seemed ludicrous because the baby's "chance" of getting it turned out to be 100% (see

Table 16-3 Risks of Psychiatric Medications in Pregnant Women

	Risks to Fetus	Risks to Mother
Continue Medication	Teratogenesis Complications at delivery Long-term neurobehavioral sequelae	
Stop Medication	Mother's untreated psychiatric disorder may harm fetus and baby	Increases chances of relapse or recurrence of her psychiatric disorder

Lithium and Pregnancy for further discussion). The following section will include the FDA's categories for drug use in pregnancy, reviews of specific psychiatric medications (e.g., SSRIs, lithium), consideration of the mother's risk for relapse and the severity of her disorder, and discussion with patients regarding the risk and benefits of medications.

FDA's Categories for Drug Use in Pregnancy

The categories used by the FDA are not very helpful in decisions about medications to use or avoid during pregnancy. One obvious problem is that there are no psychiatric drugs in category A and only 1 in category B (i.e., bupropion); thus most psychiatric medications are either category C or D. Also, a commonly held misperception is that category B drugs are "safer" than category C drugs and category C drugs are "safer" than category D drugs. These categories are primarily based on the presence or absence of evidence and not on equally weighted evidence directly comparing drugs and risk; thus the categories do not really indicate relative safety. For example, fluoxetine is the most studied SSRI in pregnancy, and a registry was created when it was released in 1989; this database is currently the largest for any antidepressant used during pregnancy and facilitated later studies of whether neuropsychological effects occurred in the children. However, fluoxetine has a category C label because rats given 10 to 18 times the recommended dosage of fluoxetine have smaller litters. In contrast, bupropion is in category B because the animal studies showed no increase in any abnormalities and the few human studies showed no increase in teratogenesis. No registry was created when bupropion was released. While neither drug has been shown to cause teratogenic effects, the FDA's current system could incorrectly lead a clinician to switch a woman's fluoxetine to bupropion because he or she believes bupropion to be safer. The FDA is aware of these concerns and is considering revising the classification system.

SSRIs and Pregnancy

SSRIs are category C drugs, except for paroxetine, which had its label changed to a category D because of a recently reported increased risk of heart defects. Two studies have shown a doubling of the baseline risk of heart defects with paroxetine from 1% to 2%. There is also a recent report of an increased association between persistent pulmonary hypertension (PPHN) of the newborn and maternal SSRI use after week 20 of gestation. The risk for PPHN increased from 1 in 1000 (0.1%) to between 6 and 12 in 1000 (0.6%-1.2%). In other words, about 99% of women exposed to an SSRI late in pregnancy will deliver an infant unaffected by PPHN. As previously noted, fluoxetine is the most studied SSRI and is considered the "safest" in pregnancy based on that database. There is the additional risk that the newborn baby may show increased muscle tone or appear jittery. These symptoms are transient and self-limited and are considered to be secondary to the SSRI or the abrupt decrease of the SSRI in the newborn at birth.

Lithium and Pregnancy

Lithium was released shortly after thalidomide and was closely watched for any abnormalities with a birth registry. When an increase in Ebstein anomaly was reported from the registry, there was a swift reaction from clinicians to avoid lithium during early pregnancy. Further study reveals that the baseline risk of 0.005% (1 in 20,000 births) increases to 0.1% (1 in 1000 births) in mothers receiving lithium. By using the change in absolute risk, the number needed to harm (NNH) is over 1000 births with lithium to get 1 additional case of Ebstein anomaly. The risk of a recurrence of bipolar disorder with cessation of lithium is about 55%, and if lithium is continued, the relapse rate during pregnancy is 0% to 10%. Using these percentages, the NNH by stopping lithium is 2. This example graphically illustrates why most psychiatrists recommend continuing lithium during pregnancy for women who have significant bipolar I disorder.

The Mother's Risk for Relapse and the Severity of Illness

The greater the likelihood of relapse or recurrence of the mother's psychiatric disorder and the greater the severity of the mother's psychiatric disorder when symptomatic, the stronger the indication to continue medications during pregnancy. Typically, clinicians consider the risks of the psychiatric disorder in terms of morbidity for the mother. However, there is potentially significant morbidity and harm to the fetus or baby and other children (if present) when the mother's psychiatric disorder recurs. Obvious examples are suicide or dangerous behaviors associated with mania or psychosis (e.g., substance abuse, impulsive acts) that clearly could hurt the fetus. Less obvious problems include decreased prenatal care, neglect of other children in the household, and decreased mother-infant bonding in the postpartum period. Furthermore, maternal depression and anxiety during pregnancy have been associated with resultant intrauterine growth retardation and premature birth. The clinician should fully assess past suicidality, hospitalizations, and substance abuse when evaluating the severity of the mother's psychiatric disorder. The risk for relapse or recurrence is mostly related to the number of previous episodes; the greater the number of episodes, the greater the likelihood of relapse and recurrence.

The Discussion of Risk with Women of Childbearing Years

The earlier the clinician discusses with the patient the potential impact of medications during pregnancy, the better. Generally, before a woman of childbearing years is given any medication, even if she is not contemplating pregnancy, there should be a full discussion of the risks and benefits of the medication and its potential effects on the fetus should she become pregnant. Having these conversations when the patient is already pregnant narrows the choices for the patient. Noting sexual activity and contraception methods is also important because they influence the likelihood of pregnancy.

Noting the severity of symptoms the mother has had with prior psychiatric episodes is crucial in this process. Particular weight is given to suicide attempts, need for hospitalization, psychosis, and mania. Patients with milder symptoms and long periods in remission will have less risk if decompensation occurs. A psychiatric consultation should be obtained if there are any questions regarding the diagnosis or need for medications.

It is particularly important to develop a plan should symptoms exacerbate. In cases of significant bipolar disorder or depression with psychotic features, the use of electroconvulsive therapy (ECT) should be discussed. ECT is the fastest working treatment for reduction of manic or depressive symptoms and is safe in pregnancy. Psychiatric consultation is strongly recommended in any patient whose mood disorder is accompanied by psychotic symptoms.

Postpartum Disorders

Most general clinicians will share the management of pregnant patients with obstetricians. However, many women in the postpartum period may only be followed by their general clinicians. This is especially true after spontaneous abortions and other terminations of pregnancy.

Postpartum mood disorders, though labeled separately, probably represent a spectrum of disorders (see Table 16-4). Postpartum blues or "baby blues" are very common and normal and are often mistaken for postpartum depression. Early postpartum depression and baby blues have the same symptoms of mood lability, anxiety, and depressed mood. However, postpartum depression will continue to advance in severity, and the blues spontaneously resolve without treatment within a week. The anxiety in postpartum depression takes on an obsessive quality usually focused on the infant. Puerperal psychosis is rare and comes on quickly after delivery; it constitutes a psychiatric emergency. Organic causes of psychosis, including Sheehan syndrome and thyroid disorders, should be considered and ruled out early when psychosis is present in the postpartum period.

Table 16-4 Classification of Postpartum Mood Disorders

Disorder	Prevalence	Onset	Characteristic Symptoms
Postpartum blues	30%-85%	Within first week	Mood lability, tearfulness, insomnia, anxiety
Postpartum depression	10%-15%	Usually insidious, within first 2 to 3 months	Depressed mood, excessive anxiety, insomnia
Puerperal psychosis	0.1%-0.2%	Usually within first 2 to 4 weeks	Agitation and irritability, depressed mood or euphoria, delusions, depersonalization, disorganized behavior

Treatment for postpartum depression follows the same approach as major depression. However, a major consideration for nursing mothers is that antidepressants are excreted into breast milk and will be subsequently ingested by a nursing infant. In some cases the infant may show side effects of the antidepressant, but in most cases no effects are noticed. The use of psychiatric medications in nursing mothers is discussed in the following section.

Lactation and Psychiatric Medications

Women who need to take a psychiatric medication during the postpartum period may want to breast-feed their infants, but evidence to guide the decision is limited. What is known is that all psychotropic medications pass into breast milk by passive diffusion. For most medications, the following properties tend to increase diffusion of the drug into breast milk: less protein-binding, more lipid-solubility, and more basic. The infant's physiology affects the absorption and metabolism of drugs, too. Infants less than 6 months old have prolonged gastric emptying and higher gastric pH; both these factors can increase degradation of the drug. Liver enzymes develop at different rates. Premature infants take the longest to develop a mature liver enzyme system. The psychiatric drugs that have at least limited data include tricyclic antidepressants (TCAs), SSRIs, benzodiazepines, and the mood stabilizers lithium, carbamazepine, and divalproex. Of these drugs, TCAs and SSRIs are probably the "safest" but by no means can be said to be risk free. Generally speaking, SSRIs can cause significant toxicity in adults, and infants are even more vulnerable.

For the mother who truly needs a psychiatric medication and wants to breast-feed her infant, the following guidelines are useful:

- Use only one agent (i.e., monotherapy) if possible.
- Use the lowest effective dose.
- Add psychotherapy and other nonpharmacological interventions (e.g., exercise, sleep hygiene, good nutrition) to medications.
- Time breast-feeding to when drug levels are at their lowest (i.e., right before taking the next dosage of medication) and store that breast milk for other feedings.
- Consider "pump and dump" for times when the drug level is highest and use stored breast milk during those times.

Perimenopause and Menopause

Symptoms around the time of menopause are physical and psychiatric. Hot flushes, diminished concentration, fatigue, and insomnia constitute the major physical symptoms of menopause. Irritability, emotional lability, and depressed feelings constitute the major psychiatric symptoms. There is a large degree of overlap between the symptoms of perimenopause and major depression, but, in general, new-onset depression is not typically associated with menopause. However, recent large prospective studies indicate that if new-onset major depression does occur, it tends to occur in the beginning of the menopausal transition when the variation in hormonal levels is the greatest (1,2). In addition, the evidence is very clear that if a woman has a past history of major depression, PMDD, or a peripartum psychiatric disorder, then she has an increased risk of developing a new episode of depression during the menopausal transition.

There is some evidence to support the treatment of depressive symptoms of perimenopause with estrogens. These studies are short term (i.e., 12 to 16 weeks) but show positive results (3). Methodologically, these are difficult studies to blind because estrogens are so obvious in their effective treatment of the physical symptoms of menopause, particularly the hot flushes. Nonetheless, women with significant symptoms of perimenopause, which include depressive symptoms, will probably benefit from a short course of estrogen replacement if not contraindicated for other reasons (e.g., history of breast cancer). Other approaches that target the sleep disturbances frequently associated with hot flushes are also effective and carry significantly less risk than hormonal therapies. The major task for the clinician is to determine if there are enough symptoms and dysfunction to meet criteria for a major depressive episode (i.e., a disorder) or if there are only a few symptoms that do not meet the threshold of a major mood disorder. Symptomatic treatment and close follow-up are indicated in the latter. However, if a woman meets the criteria for new-onset or recurrent major depression, then the most appropriate treatment is an antidepressant.

KEY POINTS

ADULT ADD

- The diagnosis of adult ADD or ADHD requires the diagnosis of childhood ADD or ADHD.
- ADD and ADHD symptom categories are hyperactivity, inattention, and impulsivity.
- The ratio of boys to girls with ADD or ADHD is 3 to 1, but the ratio of men to women with ADD or ADHD is 1 to 1.
- Most adult patients with inattention have a diagnosis other than ADD.
- Response to treatment with a stimulant does not confirm the diagnosis of ADD or ADHD.
- If a comorbid disorder is present that can cause inattention, it should be treated first before initiating stimulants.
- Both stimulants and nonstimulants are effective.
- Stimulants should not be given to patients with a history of substance abuse.

EATING DISORDERS

- Eating-disordered behaviors are much more common than full-criteria eating disorders defined by the DSM-IV.
- Anorexia nervosa (AN) is characterized by voluntary restriction of caloric intake and is the least common and most severe eating disorder.
- Bulimia nervosa (BN) is characterized by binge eating and compensatory "purging" activities (e.g., vomiting, excessive exercising, and abusing diuretics and laxatives) and is more common and generally less severe than AN.
- Binge-eating disorder (BED) is characterized by binge-eating behaviors but no compensatory measures (as in BN), and it is probably more common and more likely to spontaneously resolve than either AN or BN.
- Clinical assessment of a patient's eating behaviors should include an evaluation of nutrition, specific eating behaviors, and the psychological underpinnings (e.g., distorted body image).
- Distortion of body image is the most pervasive psychological feature across all eating disorders.

WOMEN'S HEALTH

- Premenstrual symptoms are very common, but PMDD is not.
- Premenstrual psychiatric symptoms are more likely to represent the worsening of another psychiatric disorder (e.g., dysthymia) than PMDD.
- Potential risks and benefits of medications during pregnancy should be considered in all women of childbearing years.
- Discussion and subsequent documentation regarding potential risks and benefits to the fetus or baby and mother should occur before prescribing any medication to a pregnant patient.
- Pregnancy neither protects nor promotes psychiatric illness.
- Postpartum psychiatric disorders either represent a recurrence of an existing psychiatric disorder or a new onset of one.
- All psychiatric drugs passively diffuse into the mother's breast milk.
- Perimenopause increases the chances of a recurrence of depression.
- A new onset of a major depressive episode most often occurs early in the menopausal transition.

REFERENCES

1. Cohen LS, Soares CN, Vitonis AF, et al. Risk for new onset of depression during the menopausal transition: the Harvard study of moods and cycles. *Arch Gen Psychiatry.* 2006;63(4):385-390.
2. Freeman EW, Sammel MD, Lin H, et al. Associations of hormones and menopausal status with depressed mood in women with no history of depression. *Arch Gen Psychiatry.* 2006;63(4):375-382.
3. Cohen LS, Soares CN, Poitras JR, et al. Short-term use of estradiol for depression in perimenopausal and postmenopausal women: a preliminary report. *Am J Psychiatry.* 2003;160(8):1519-1522.

KEY REFERENCES

Altshuler LL, Cohen LS, Moline ML, et al. Expert consensus panel for depression in women. The expert consensus guideline series. Treatment of depression in women. *Postgrad Med.* 2001;(Spec No):1-107.

American Psychiatric Association. Treatment of patients with eating disorders, third edition. *Am J Psychiatry.* 2006;163(7):4-54.

Biederman J, Faraone SV, Milberger S, et al. Predictors of persistence and remission of ADHD into adolescence: results from a four year prospective follow-up study. *J Am Acad Child Adolesc Psychiatry.* 1996;35:343-351.

Biederman J, Mick E, Faraone SV. Age-dependent decline of symptoms of attention deficit hyperactivity disorder: impact of remission definition and symptom type. *Am J Psychiatry.* 2000;157:816-818.

Bulik CM, Sullivan PF, Kendler KS. An empirical study of the classification of eating disorders. *Am J Psychiatry.* 2000;157:886-895.

Claudino AM, Hay P, Lima MS, et al. Antidepressants for anorexia nervosa. *Cochrane Database Syst Rev.* 2006; 1:CD004365.

Cohen LS, Altshuler LL, Harlow BL, et al. Relapse of major depression during pregnancy in women who maintain or discontinue antidepressant treatment. *JAMA.* 2006;295:499-507.

Cohen LS, Soares CN, Joffe H. Diagnosis and management of mood disorders during the menopausal transition. *Am J Med.* 2005;118:935.

Di Giulio G, Reissing ED. Premenstrual dysphoric disorder: prevalence, diagnostic considerations, and controversies. *J Psychosom Obstet Gynaecol.* 2006;27(4):201-210.

Faraone SV, Biederman J, Feighner JA, et al. Assessing symptoms of attention deficit hyperactivity disorder in children and adults: which is more valid? *J Consult Clin Psychol.* 2000;68:830-842.

Faraone SV, Biederman J, Spencer T, et al. Diagnosing adult attention deficit hyperactivity disorder: are late onset and subthreshold diagnoses valid? *Am J Psychiatry.* 2006;163(10):1720-1729.

Godart NT, Perdereau F, Rein Z, et al. Comorbidity studies of eating disorders and mood disorders. Critical review of the literature. *J Affect Disord.* 2007;97(1-3):37-49.

Mannucci E, Rotella F, Ricca V, et al. Eating disorders in patients with type 1 diabetes: a meta-analysis. *J Endocrinol Invest.* 2005 May;28(5):417-419.

McGough JJ, Barkley RA. Diagnostic controversies in adult attention deficit hyperactivity disorder. *Am J Psychiatry.* 2004;161(11):1948-1956.

Moses-Kolko EL, Roth EK. Antepartum and postpartum depression: healthy mom, healthy baby. *J Am Med Womens Assoc.* 2004;59(3):181-191.

Pritts SD, Susman J. Diagnosis of eating disorders in primary care. *Am Fam Physician.* 2003;67:297-304,311-312.

Wilens TE. Attention-deficit/hyperactivity disorder and the substance use disorders: the nature of the relationship, subtypes at risk, and treatment issues. *Psych Clin N Am.* 2004;27(2):283-301.

Wyatt KM, Dimmock PW, O'Brien PM. Selective serotonin reuptake inhibitors for premenstrual syndrome. *Cochrane Database Syst Rev.* 2002;4:CD001396.

Appendix

■ Patient Medication Guide

Medication Guide
**Antidepressant Medicines, Depression and Other Serious
Mental Illnesses, and Suicidal Thoughts or Actions**

Read the Medication Guide that comes with you or your family member's antidepressant medicine. This Medication Guide is only about the risk of suicidal thoughts and actions with antidepressant medicines. **Talk to your, or your family member's, healthcare provider about:**

- all risks and benefits of treatment with antidepressant medicines
- all treatment choices for depression or other serious mental illness

What is the most important information I should know about antidepressant medicines, depression and other serious mental illnesses, and suicidal thoughts or actions?

1. Antidepressant medicines may increase suicidal thoughts or actions in some children, teenagers, and young adults when the medicine is first started.

2. Depression and other serious mental illnesses are the most important causes of suicidal thoughts and actions. Some people may have a particularly high risk of having suicidal thoughts or actions. (These include people who have (or have a family history of) bipolar illness also called manic-depressive illness) or suicidal thoughts or actions.

3. How can I watch for and try to prevent suicidal thoughts and actions in myself or a family member?

- Pay close attention to any changes, especially sudden changes, in mood, behaviors, thoughts, or feelings. This is very important when an antidepressant medicine is first started or when the dose is changed.
- Call the healthcare provider right away to report new or sudden changes in mood, behavior, thoughts, or feelings.
- Keep all follow-up visits with the healthcare provider as scheduled. Call the healthcare provider between visits as needed, especially if you have concerns about symptoms.

Call a healthcare provider right away if you or your family member has any of the following symptoms, especially if they are new, worsen, or worry you:

- thoughts about suicide or dying
- attempts to commit suicide
- new or worse depression
- new or worse anxiety
- feeling very agitated or restless
- panic attacks
- trouble sleeping (insomnia)
- new or worse irritability
- acting aggressive, being angry, or violent
- acting on dangerous impulses
- an extreme increase in activity and talking (mania)
- other unusual changes in behavior or mood

What else do I need to know about antidepressant medicines?

- **Never stop an antidepressant medicine without first talking to a healthcare provider.** Stopping an antidepressant medicine suddenly can cause other symptoms.
- **Antidepressants are medicines used to treat depression and other illnesses.** It is important to discuss all the risks of treating depression and also the risks of not treating it. Patients and their families or other caregivers should discuss all treatment choices with the healthcare provider, not just the use of antidepressants.
- **Antidepressant medicines have other side effects.** Talk to the healthcare provider about the side effects of the medicine prescribed for you or your family member.
- **Antidepressant medicines can interact with other medicines.** Know all of the medicines that you or your family member takes. Keep a list of all medicines to show the healthcare provider. Do not start new medicines without first checking with your healthcare provider.
- **Not all antidepressant medicines prescribed for children are FDA approved for use in children.** Talk to your child's healthcare provider for more information.

This Medication Guide has been approved by the U.S. Food and Drug Administration for all antidepressants.

Revised 21 June 2007

■ MAOI Diet

Foods to Avoid

- Alcoholic beverages (especially red wines and "yeasty" beers)
- Bean curd
- Broad (fava) bean pods
- Cheese (cream cheese and cottage cheese have no detectable level of tyramine)
- Smoked fish or meat
- Sausage, bologna, pepperoni, and salami
- Ginseng
- Protein extracts
- Sauerkraut
- Shrimp Paste
- Yeast

Foods to Use with Caution

- Avocados
- Caffeine
- Chocolate
- Dairy products (cream, sour cream, cottage cheese, cream cheese, yogurt, or milk)
- Nuts
- Raspberries
- Soy sauce
- Spinach

Foods with Insufficient Evidence for Restriction

- Anchovies
- Beetroot
- Chips with vinegar
- Cockles
- Corn, sweet
- Cucumbers
- Egg, boiled
- Figs, canned
- Fish, canned
- Mushrooms
- Pineapple, fresh
- Raisins
- Salad dressings
- Snails
- Tomato juice

- Wild game
- Worcestershire sauce
- Yeast-leavened bread

References

Gardner DM, Shulman KI, Walker SE. The making of a user-friendly MAOI diet. *J Clin Psychiatry.* 1996;57:99-104

Shulman KI, Walker SE. Refining the MAOI diet: tyramine content of pizzas and soy products. *J Clin Psychiatry.* 1999;60:191-193.

Foods interacting with MAOI inhibitors. *Med Lett Drug Ther.* 1989;31:11-12.

Ayd FJ. Diet and monoamine oxidase inhibitors (MAOIs): an update. *Int Drug Ther Newslett.* 1986; 21:19-20.

Gilman AG, Goodman LS, Rall TW, et al, eds. *Goodman and Gilman's The Pharmacological Basis of Therapeutics.* 7th ed. New York: Macmillan, 1985.

Lippman SB, Nash K. Monoamine oxidase inhibitor update. Potential adverse food and drug interactions. *Drug Safety.* 1990;5:195-204.

McCabe BJ. Dietary tyramine and other pressor amines in MAOI regimens: a review. *J Am Diet Assoc.* 1986;86:1059-1064.

Zisook S. A clinical overview of monoamine oxidase inhibitors. *Psychosomatics.* 1985;26:240-251.

Index